Models of Viral Hepatitis

Kompetenznetz Hepatitis

Monographs in Virology

Vol. 25

Series Editor

H.W. Doerr *Frankfurt*

KARGER

Models of Viral Hepatitis

Volume Editors

Fritz von Weizsäcker *Freiburg*
Michael Roggendorf *Essen*

27 figures, 1 in color, and 5 tables, 2005

KARGER

Basel · Freiburg · Paris · London · New York ·
Bangalore · Bangkok · Singapore · Tokyo · Sydney

Fritz von Weizsäcker
Medizinische Universitätsklinik
Abteilung Innere Medizin II
Hugstetterstrasse 55
D–79106 Freiburg (Germany)

Michael Roggendorf
Institut für Virologie
Universitätsklinikum Essen
Hufelandstrasse 55
D–45122 Essen (Germany)

Library of Congress Cataloging-in-Publication Data

Models of viral hepatitis / volume editors, Fritz von Weizsäcker, Michael Roggendorf.
p. ; cm. – (Monographs in virology ; v. 25)
Includes bibliographical references and index.
ISBN 3-8055-7809-1 (hard cover : alk. paper)
1. Hepatitis, Viral–Animal models. I. Weizsäcker, Fritz von.
II. Roggendorf, Michael. III. Series.
[DNLM: 1. Disease Models, Animal. 2. Hepatitis, Viral, Human.
3. Hepatitis, Viral, Animal. WC 536 M689 2005]
QR201.H46M63 2005
616.3′623–dc22

2004020576

Bibliographic Indices. This publication is listed in bibliographic services, including Current Contents® and Index Medicus.

Drug Dosage. The authors and the publisher have exerted every effort to ensure that drug selection and dosage set forth in this text are in accord with current recommendations and practice at the time of publication. However, in view of ongoing research, changes in government regulations, and the constant flow of information relating to drug therapy and drug reactions, the reader is urged to check the package insert for each drug for any change in indications and dosage and for added warnings and precautions. This is particularly important when the recommended agent is a new and/or infrequently employed drug.

www.karger.com
Printed in Switzerland on acid-free paper by Reinhardt Druck, Basel
ISSN 0077–0965
ISBN 3–8055–7809–1

Contents

Foreword

Viral hepatitis B or C is the most common cause of chronic liver disease worldwide and accounts for about 80% of all hepatocellular carcinoma cases. Despite significant progress in our understanding of viral hepatitis, effective treatment options are still unavailable for a large number of patients and many basic and clinical problems remain unresolved. For example, little is known about the cellular factors mediating HBV and HCV entry and uncoating. Furthermore, the contribution of innate and adaptive immune responses in the early phase of infection for viral clearance and persistence is not fully understood. To address these and other important issues, such as drug testing, immunomodulatory strategies and HCC pathogenesis, animal models and cell-based tools are of central importance. Several animal models have been established for hepadnaviral infection. Each of them contributes to the understanding of pathogenesis in a specific way. For example, much has been learned about the immune response to mammalian hepadnaviral infection and development of hepatocellular carcinoma in the woodchuck model, while the duck model has been extensively utilized for assessing antiviral strategies. Regarding HCV, the chimpanzee is the only reliable animal model thus far. Nevertheless, the development of the replicon system has yielded a wealth of important insights in HCV replication and virus-cell interactions.

In 2002 the German network of excellence for viral hepatitis (Hep-Net) set out to promote horizontal networking among research groups working on models of hepatitis B and C. The aim was to accelerate the translation of basic viral research into clinical application by strengthening cooperations and by joining resources of the respective models. As a first step, a HepNet workshop on models of viral hepatitis was held in February 2003 at the Conference Centre of Elmau, Germany. Leading experts reported new scientific results and evolving methods in various animal and in vitro models of viral hepatitis. The present monograph summarizes the state of the art in these different model systems.

We hope that this unique synopsis may help understand the technical challenges and specific strengths of each model and may stimulate interested researchers to participate in the network. The editors are grateful to Glaxo Smith Kline Beecham, Abbott GmbH, and Gilead Sciences GmbH, whose support made the publication of this book possible.

F. von Weizsäcker
M. Roggendorf

von Weizsäcker F, Roggendorf M (eds): Models of Viral Hepatitis.
Monogr Virol. Basel, Karger, 2005, vol 25, pp 1–24

The Woodchuck: A Model for Immunopathogenesis and Therapy of Hepadnaviral Infection

M. Roggendorf, M. Lu

Institute of Virology, University of Essen, Germany

Since the discovery of hepatitis B virus (HBV) in the 1960s, a number of genetically closely related viruses have been described. Woodchuck hepatitis virus (WHV), which infects Eastern woodchucks (*Marmota monax*) (fig. 1), was discovered in 1978 [68] followed by duck hepatitis virus; both were found to be closely related to HBV [51]. WHV was classified as a member of the genus orthohepadnavirus of the family hepadnaviridae [20]. However, this virus differs from HBV in several aspects, e.g. regulation of transcription [14]. The family hepadnaviridae is still growing in the recent years [39, 77]. Infections of woodchucks with WHV have been shown to be endemic in the Mid-Atlantic States of the USA, e.g. Delaware, Maryland, Pennsylvania, whereas in the State of New York and New England, woodchucks are rarely infected with WHV. The molecular characterization of WHV and experimental infection of woodchucks with WHV has been of value in modeling several aspects of hepadnavirus infection in humans. Many questions of hepadnavirus infection have been addressed in this model, e.g. natural course of infection [9, 28, 33, 53], immunopathogenesis [53, 54, 56, 57, 59, 75, 76], host and viral factors associated to development of chronicity [8, 60, 76], development of hepatocellular carcinoma (HCC) [18, 72], and rise and significance of viral mutants in acute and chronic infection [2–4, 42, 47, 70, 81, 84, 86]. From a medical point of view, the woodchuck model has been used to develop new strategies for prevention of infection [21, 45] and therapy of chronic hepadnaviral infection including: nucleoside analogues [10, 11, 22, 32, 35–37, 40, 52, 64, 85, 89, 90], non-nucleoside analogues [1, 15], therapeutic vaccination [29, 46, 49, 58], and gene therapeutic approaches for treatment of HCC [65]. Liver transplantation has recently been established for woodchucks to study early events in reinfection and adoptive

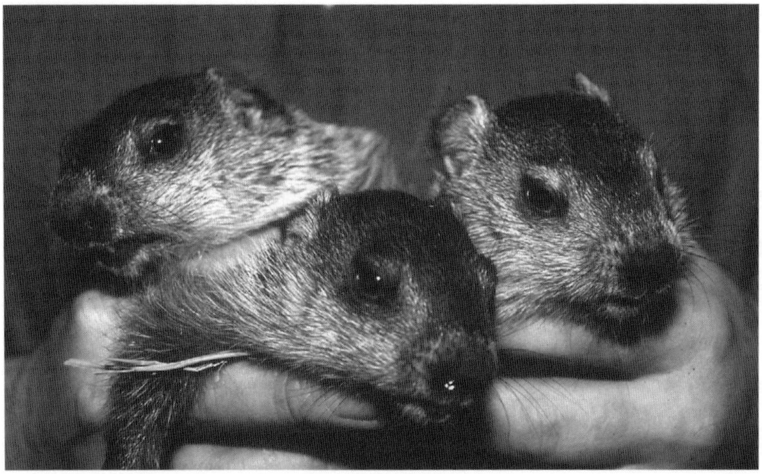

Fig. 1. Six-week-old woodchucks.

immune transfer [12, 13]. Previous reviews covered the natural history of WHV infection [73], etiology of HCC [72], antiviral treatment by nucleoside analogues [71, 87, 88], and pathogenesis of hepadnaviral infection [53]. Lately, significant progress has been made in this model of hepadnavirus natural infection which demonstrates that non-cytotoxic and cytolytic antiviral immune responses are needed for elimination of the virus from hepatocytes or to at least control viral replication. This review therefore focuses on the immunopathogenesis of WHV infection. We describe here the recent development of tools to study humoral and cellular immune response to WHV and adoptive immunotransfer after liver transplantation to treat chronic WHV infection. These new insights into the immune response to WHV will enable the development of new strategies to treat chronic HBV infection.

The Immune System of the Woodchuck

The woodchuck is an ideal model for hepadnavirus infection in humans as WHV infection in woodchucks results in a number of different outcomes which are similar to HBV infection in humans, ranging from a subclinical or acute transient infection to chronic infection progressing to HCC. Unfortunately, no inbred animals are available so far to standardize infection experiments. For the understanding of the underlying mechanisms responsible for different outcomes of infection, detailed in vivo studies on humoral and cellular immune response to WHV are required. Assays for antigen and antibody detection have been

Table 1. Cloned cytokines of woodchuck

	Size	Homology (aa) human/mouse, %	Biologically active	Accession no.	Group (first author)
TNF-α	233 aa	80/84	+	Y14137	Lohrengel, 1998 [43], Lohrengel, 2000 [44]
IFN-γ	166 aa	60/43	+	Y14138	Lohrengel, 1998 [43], Lu, 2002 [48]
IFN-α	167 aa	62/58	+	AAG27516 AAK19944	Sallucci, 2002 [67]
IL-2	Partial			AF082496	Lu [unpubl. results]
IL-4	Partial			AF082495	Lu [unpubl. results]
IL-6	207 aa	49/46	ND	Y14139	Lohrengel, 1998 [43]
IL-10	178 aa	80/72	ND	AF012909	Li, 2000 [41]
IL-12 p35	223 aa	62/51	+	X97018	Garcia-Navarro, 2002 [21]
IL-12 p40	325 aa	78/65	+	X97019	Garcia-Navarro, 2002 [21]
IL-15	192 aa	79/70	+	AY426605	Wang [76]
GMCSF	138 aa	63/49	+	AF255734	Wu, 2001 [88]
LT-α	202 aa	78/80	+	AF095586	Li, 2000 [41]
LT-β	306 aa	67/69	ND	AF095587	Li, 2000 [41]
Fas ligand	Partial		ND	AF152368	Hodgson, 1999 [31]

available for many years [66]. However, until recently, only little information has been available about components of the woodchuck immune system and the cellular immune response.

In recent years a number of cytokines and surface markers of immune cells have been characterized. Proteins related to immune response like antigen processing (TAP-1, TAP-2) and presentation, e.g. MHC class I and class II, proteins involved in signal transduction, and cell surface markers like CD3, CD54, and CD8 present of cells of the immune system, have been cloned and sequenced. The components of the woodchuck immune system characterized at the molecular level so far are summarized in tables 1 and 2. In general, cDNA fragments were amplified by reversed transcription polymerase chain reaction with RNAs from woodchuck lymphocytes. Primers were designed according to aligned sequences and chosen from regions well conserved among human and other mammalian species.

Cytokines

The complete sequence of tumor necrosis factor-α (TNF-α) [41, 43], interferon (IFN)-α [67], IFN-γ [43], interleukin (IL)-6 [43], IL-10 [42], IL-12 [21]

Table 2. Clonal cell surface marker and other genes related to the woodchuck immune system

Gene	Sequence information	Homology (aa) human/mouse, %	Accession no.	Group (first author)
CD3-γ	Partial		AF082493	Nakamuro, 2001 [62]
CD3-ε	Partial		AF232727	Michalak, 2000 [59]
CD4	455 aa		AF082497	Zhou, 1999 [86], Fiedler [unpubl. results]
CD8	Partial		AF082499	Zhou, 1999 [86]
CD28	221 aa	76/74	AF130427	Yang, 2003 [83]
CTLA-4	223 aa	86/85	AF130428	Yang, 2003 [83]
MHC-I (*Mamo-I*)	359 aa	81–83/78–79	AF146091 etc.	Yang, 2003 [82]
MHC-II (WLA)	266 aa	87/80		Viazov [unpubl. results]
β_2-Microglobulin	Partial		AF232726	Michalak, 2000 [59]
TAP-1	Partial		AF232724	Michalak, 2000 [59]
TAP-2	Partial		AF232725	Michalak, 2000 [59]
2′,5′-Oligoadenylate synthetase	Partial		AF082498	Zhou, 1999 [86]
Stat4	Partial		AY177676	Wang, 2003 [76]
Stat6	Partial		AY177677	Wang, 2003 [76]
T-bet	Partial		AY177675	Wang, 2003 [76]
GATA-binding protein 3	Partial		AY177678	Wang, 2003 [76]
PemI	Partial		AY494083	Fourel, 1994 [19]
Perforin	Partial		AF298158	Hodgson, 1999 [31]
Tumor suppressor p53	391 aa	86/77	AJ001022	Feitelson, 1997 [17]

and IL-15 [76], GMCSF [80], lymphotoxin (LT)-α and LT-β [42] were obtained. Partial sequences of IL-2, IL-4, Fas ligand [31] and others were cloned. The length and homology of woodchuck cytokines to human and mouse cytokines are given in table 1. In general, the woodchuck genes are more closely related to the human than to the mouse counterpart. The structure of woodchuck cytokines as compared to human cytokines seems to be well conserved, e.g. the comparison of WHV TNF-α to the human sequence demonstrates that two cysteine residues cys69 and cys101 that are known to be involved in an intermolecular disulfide bridge are conserved. Other amino acid residues like leu29, arg32, ala143, and ser145 which were found to be important for receptor binding of the human protein are also conserved in the woodchuck TNF-α [43]. For IFN-α it could also be shown that four cysteine residues which form intramolecular disulfide bridges are conserved [67].

TNF-α, IFN-α, IFN-γ, IL-12, and LT-α have been tested for their biological activities. The entire ORF of IFN-α was cloned under control of the CMV promoter into the expression vector PVIJ [67]. Supernatants of HeLa cells transfected with this construct protected woodchuck cells from a VSV-induced cytopathic effect. The biological action of IFN-α was also demonstrated by induction of expression at MXA protein. Finally, the biological activity of IFN-α was tested in WHV-infected woodchuck hepatocytes. Woodchuck IFN-α reduced WHV surface antigen expression in a dose-dependent fashion [67].

The biological activity of TNF-α and LT-α was tested in a cytotoxicity assay using woodchuck A2 cells. The specific activities for both woodchuck cytokines TNF-α and LT-α were significantly higher in woodchuck cells than in mouse L9–9B and human HepG2 cells [42, 43].

We expressed recombinant woodchuck IFN-γ (wIFN-γ) in *Escherichia coli* and mammalian cells. The biological activity of IFN-γ was demonstrated by experiments showing that recombinant wIFN-γ protected woodchuck cells against infection with murine encephalomyocarditis virus in a species-specific manner. It up-regulates the mRNA level of the woodchuck major histocompatibility complex class I (*Mamo-I*) heavy chain in permanent woodchuck WH12/6 cells and regulated differentially the gene expression [48]. However, the level of the replication intermediates and specific RNAs of WHV in persistently WHV-infected primary woodchuck hepatocytes did not change despite treatment with 1,000 U of wIFN-γ/ml or with a combination of wIFN-γ and woodchuck wTNF-α (fig. 2). Rabbit antibodies to wIFN-γ were able to block the biological activity of IFN-γ.

Cell Surface Markers

Characterization of T-cell markers is a prerequisite to define T-cell subpopulations and to functionally analyze these cells in the course of acute and chronic infection. By designing primers chosen from regions conserved among humans and other mammalian species, fragments of CD3, CD8, and the complete sequence of CD4 have been cloned (table 2). The complete coding region of woodchuck CD4 has a length of 1,365 bp encoding a protein of 455aa [Fiedler, unpubl. results]. The cDNAs of woodchuck CD28 and cytotoxic T-lymphocyte-associated antigen 4 (CTLA-4) have been cloned and sequenced [83]. These two molecules are known to play important roles for the regulation of T-cell activation by delivering the costimulation signals. Woodchuck CD28 showed a similarity of 70–80% to its mammalian homologues according to the deduced amino acid sequences. Woodchuck CTLA-4 has a higher similarity of 74% to the corresponding mammalian CTLA-4 molecules. The strict conservation of critical amino acid residues like cysteine and asparagine residues in woodchuck CD28 and CTLA-4 suggests that both molecules may structurally resemble their human or mouse homologues. A hexapeptide motif MYPPPY that has been supposed to be essential for the interaction with CD80 is present in both woodchuck CD28 and CTLA-4 [83].

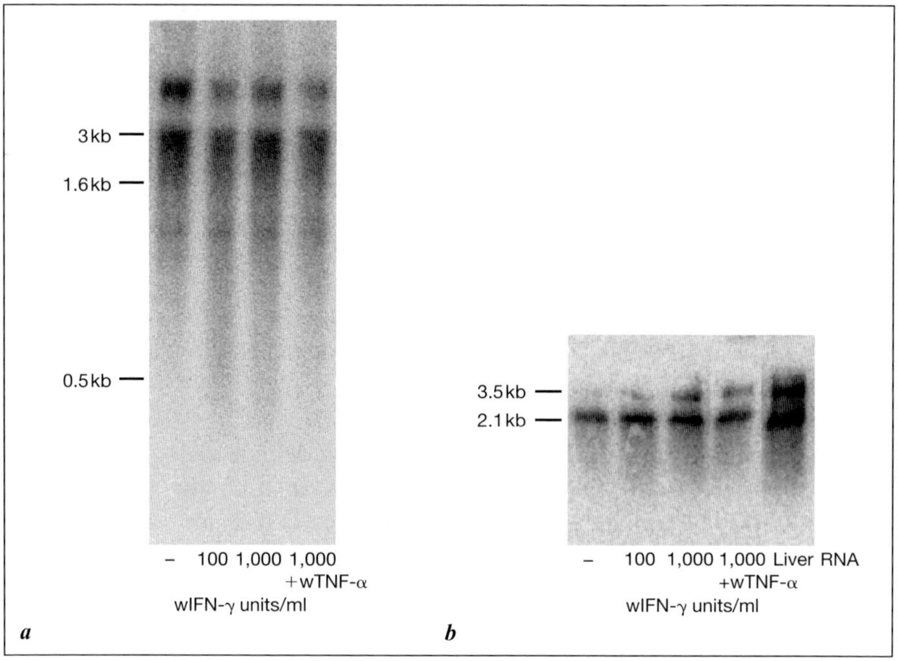

Fig. 2. WHV replication and gene expression in persistently WHV-infected primary woodchuck hepatocytes treated with 0, 100 and 1,000 U of wIFN-γ/ml or in combination with 100 U of wTNF-α/ml at day 7. Dilutions of the supernatant of peWHIG-transfected BKH cells (100 U of wIFN-γ/ml) or wPBMC culture supernatant (1,000 U of wIFN-γ/ml) were used for experiments. For control (–), the supernatant of BKH cells transfected with the control vector pcDNA3 was used at a dilution of 1:10. ***a*** WHV replication intermediates in primary woodchuck hepatocytes detected by Southern blotting. ***b*** WHV-specific mRNAs detected by Northern blotting. An RNA sample from WHV-infected woodchuck liver tissues was used as a standard.

Sequence information of woodchuck CD3 [61], CD4 [87], and CD8 [88] has been used to determine the kinetics of influx of T cells into the liver. Either sequences of wIFN-α and wTNF-α were suitable to determine cytokine expression during the incubation period and acute or chronic WHV infection [28, 69]. In week 2 post-infection, an influx of CD3+ lymphocytes could be observed and reached higher levels prior to and during the recovery phase. The peak level of CD4+ and CD8+ T cells coincided with recovery. Mono- or polyclonal antibodies to CD3+, CD4+ and CD8+ of woodchuck are not available yet. One monoclonal antibody to the conserved region of CD3 from swine was found to cross-react to woodchuck lymphocytes. The antibody was used to identify T cells in the liver during acute and chronic WHV infection. During transient infection, T cells can accumulate in the liver and reach up to two-thirds of the total number of liver cells [28].

MHC Class I

The full-length cDNAs of woodchuck major histocompatibility complex class I (*Mamo-I*) genes were cloned by using cellular mRNA isolated from peripheral blood mononuclear cells and liver tissues of woodchucks. DNA sequence analysis of *Mamo-I* cDNAs revealed that the coding regions of *Mamo-I* genes were about 1,080 bp long, encoding 359 amino acid residues [83]. The deduced amino acid sequences of *Mamo-I* showed structural features like leader, α1, α2, α3, transmembrane and cytoplasmic domains, similar to the homologous ones in humans and other mammals. Analysis of five full-length clones from unrelated woodchucks indicated a polymorphism within the α1 and α2 domains of *Mamo-I* heavy chain and a high conservation within the α3 and the transmembrane/cytoplasmic domains. Amino acid residues of the α2 and α3 domains, that are supposed to be involved in the binding of MHC class I to CD8 molecule, were largely conserved among *Mamo-I* genes. Phylogenetic comparison of woodchuck MHC class I genes to other mammals indicated a close evolutionary relationship between woodchuck and squirrel MHC class I [83]. Among the 14 alleles identified so far, *Mamo-A**01 and *Mamo-A**09 were of the highest frequency of about 21.5 and 14.5%, respectively.

To prove the allelic nature of *Mamo-I* genes by classical genetics, the segregation analysis allelic diversity of *Mamo-I* in two three-generation woodchuck families consisting of 15 members was analyzed. Alleles were identified by sequencing of *Mamo-I* genes and immunoblotting of *Mamo-I* proteins after one-dimensional isoelectric focusing. A typical Mendelian segregation of *Mamo-I* gene and antigens was observed in the families studied [87]. Our study established *Mamo-A* as a classical MHC class I locus by the polymorphic and allelic nature of *Mamo-I* gene in the woodchuck. Full-length cDNA of *Mamo-I* has been transfected to mouse p815 cells and peptides bound to MHC-I eluted from the transfected p815 cells were analyzed. The potential anchor sequence of eluted peptides has been identified for *Mamo-I* [Stephanovic, unpubl. results]. This information will be used to generate peptides of WHcAg and WHsAg, which are potential epitopes for CTL in woodchuck with the *Mamo-I* allele.

MHC Class II

MHC class II sequences have also been identified. The putative protein has 266 aa and has a typical domain like signal peptide P_1Domain, β_2Domain, transmembrane and cytosolic domain. So far, 14 alleles have been identified and one of those has a high frequency of 69% in our woodchuck cohort. The overall homology of MHC clad II of woodchuck is 87% to the human analogous DRB [S. Viazov, unpubl. results].

Characterization of Specific T-Cell Immune Response to WHV in the Woodchuck

Studies on the cellular immune response to WHV were hampered for many years because of the lack of effective proliferation assays for peripheral blood mononuclear cells (PBMC). Thymidine uptake of woodchuck PBMC stimulated by mitogens or specific WHV proteins was very low as compared to other cell systems like mouse or human, though mitogen clearly induced blast formation of woodchuck cells, as confirmed by microscopy examination. Based on the negative results reported thus far, the experimental conditions were re-evaluated to measure antigen-induced PBMC proliferation [38]. The lack of incorporation of [^{3}H]-thymidine into cellular DNA by PBMC was due to the absence of expression of thymidine kinase (TK) gene in the woodchuck lymphocytes; however, the TK gene is present in the woodchuck genome and may probably be expressed in other cell types [50]. Transfection of woodchuck cells with mouse TK gene demonstrates that TK1 is transcribed and a functional TK protein can be expressed [50]. Using 2[^{3}H]-adenine as an alternative labeled nucleoside, we could demonstrate a significant incorporation into cellular DNA and partially RNA in proliferating PBMCs [54]. In addition to 2[^{3}H]-adenine, a non-radioactive proliferation assay for woodchuck PBMCs using 5-bromo-2′-deoxyuridine (BrdU) as a thymidine analogue was established [55]. However, measurement of PBMC proliferation induced by mitogens and WHV core protein (WHcAg) by the incorporation of BrdU was less sensitive as compared to the assay using 2[^{3}H]-adenine. Another alternative assay to determine T-cell proliferation was established by measuring secretion of IL-2 of activated T cells [7, 29]. In this assay, woodchuck IL-2 secreted in supernatants from stimulated PBMCs was tested in an IL-2-dependent murine cell line, CTLL-2, indicating a cross-reactivity of mouse and woodchuck IL-2. Viral proteins for in vitro stimulations were obtained by purification of WHsAg from plasma and recombinant WHcAg in *E. coli*. Using overlapping and non-overlapping peptides derived from WHcAg, a number of T-cell epitopes on WHcAg could be identified (for details, see below). These modified and optimized proliferation assays allowed to perform studies on T-cell immune response, specifically WHV proteins in acute, chronic infection, and immunized woodchucks [55]. It remained to be proven that stimulated T cells are actually CD4+ T-helper cells because of the lack of specific antibody to the woodchuck homologue of CD4. A cross-reacting anti-CD3 antibody from swine binds to these cells [54, 56]. It can be assumed that proliferating CD3+ T cells correspond to the T-helper cell population which expand under similar experimental conditions in the mouse system. Despite many efforts, demonstration of cytotoxic T cells has not been achieved for the woodchuck model. Using DNA vaccination in mice with plasmids expressing WHcAg-specific CTLs to WHcAg could be demonstrated in the mouse model [Isogawa et al., unpubl. results].

Kinetics of T-Cell Response during Incubation Period and Acute Phase of WHV Infection

Currently the major issue in pathogenesis of hepadnavirus infection is how the immune system contributes to the elimination of the virus from the liver and which viral and/or host factors determine the recovery or chronic outcome after an acute phase of hepadnavirus infection [25]. There is a controversial discussion on the contribution of cytokines secreted by NK cells, T-helper cells, and cytotoxic T cells for down-regulation of hepadnavirus replication at the early stage of acute infection [27]. At a later time point of acute infection, cytolytic function of CTLs seems to be responsible for elimination of infected hepatocytes and for the ultimate recovery from HBV infection [24, 26].

In several studies the course of WHV infection after experimental infection has been investigated either intravenously or subcutaneously. After inoculation of adult woodchucks with a medium titer of WHV (10^5–10^8), viremia can be detected at week 2 [8]. Maximal titers of WHV are observed in the serum during weeks 6–8. WHsAg and anti-WHc are detected in weeks 3–5 and 4–6 respectively. Inoculation of low titer WHV resulted in a very short and late viremia in some animals. The only marker of infection was seroconversion to anti-HBc 8–10 weeks after inoculation (Roggendorf, unpubl. results). In neonate subcutaneous infections, viremia seems to be delayed as compared to intravenous infections of adult animals [8]. Low titer infection of neonate woodchucks is also associated with a lower carrier rate [9]. The highest levels of WHV DNA always precede the peak of SDH which is a good marker of hepatocyte lysis [56]. It has been demonstrated that influx of CD8+ T cells in the liver of woodchucks reaches maximal levels when viral DNA replication and expression of core protein is already reduced [28, 30], similar to the situation during HBV infection in chimpanzees and patients. These findings indicate that noncytolytic mechanisms are involved in down-regulation of WHV replication and most probably CTLs are responsible for elimination of infected hepatocytes as was shown in chimpanzees [74, 79], in transgenic mice [26], and patients [78].

The problem of virus elimination without lysis in the majority of infected hepatocytes in a very short time window has been elucidated in a recent study by Summers et al. [69]. They used the presence of viral DNA sequences uniquely integrated into the DNA of a small fraction of infected hepatocytes as genetic markers for the population of infected cells to follow the fate of the infected cells during viral clearance. They found that after recovery from the infection there was no discernible reduction in the number of copies of integrated viral DNA in the liver, indicating that the uninfected cells of a recovered liver were derived primarily from infected cells.

Experimental infections of woodchuck provide the opportunity to study the detailed kinetics of WHV-specific T-helper cells during the early incubation phase in the peripheral blood and the liver. This has not yet been tested in chimpanzees and humans. The strength of T-helper response may be important for the clinical outcomes of infection (see below). The establishment of methods to determine T-cell proliferation [7, 38, 55, 58] has made it possible in recent years to monitor the dynamics of T-cell response to WHsAg, WHcAg and derived peptides after experimental infection during the incubation period, acute and chronic disease under well-defined conditions in detail. The response of woodchuck T cells to WHsAg recombinant WHcAg and WHcAg-derived peptides was monitored by 2[^{3}H]-adenine assay which had a higher sensitivity than that assay using BrDU incorporation.

The first T-cell responses against WHsAg were detected 3 weeks after WHV inoculation (fig. 3). The maximum T-cell responses to WHsAg occurred when WHsAg was detected in serum and decreased upon seroconversion to anti-HBs. The development of anti-WHs which is regarded as a virus-neutralizing antibody was associated with the elimination of WHsAg from the serum. These findings suggest that T-helper cell responses to WHsAg occur very early in the infection before liver damage takes place as shown by the presence of normal SDH levels in the serum. The T-helper cell response to recombinant WHV core protein was seen in week 4, generally 1 week later than HBsAg-specific T-cell responses. In independent experiments, CD4+ T cells were detected in the liver at week 3 [28]. However, it has not been determined whether these cells were specific to WHV epitopes. Similar to the early response in the WHV-infected woodchucks, an early CD4+ T-cell response could be observed during the incubation period in a limited number of patients [78]. In chimpanzee experiments, the application of anti-CD4 antibodies at week 6 did not alter the course of infection. The interpretation for this has been that T-helper cells are no longer needed after week 6. However, elimination of CD8+ T cells through a specific antibody results in a prolonged viremia in these chimpanzees. The virus was eliminated after rebound of specific CD8+ T cell, indicating that specific CD8+ T cells are essential for virus elimination [74, 79].

Mapping of T-Helper Epitopes

The T-cell responses to the peptides derived from WHcAg measured in different studies indicate that at least 10 different epitopes located throughout the entire core protein are recognized in woodchucks. Different subsets of WHc epitopes were recognized by different animals (at least 4 in each animal) during acute self-limited infection. The large number of epitopes may be explained by

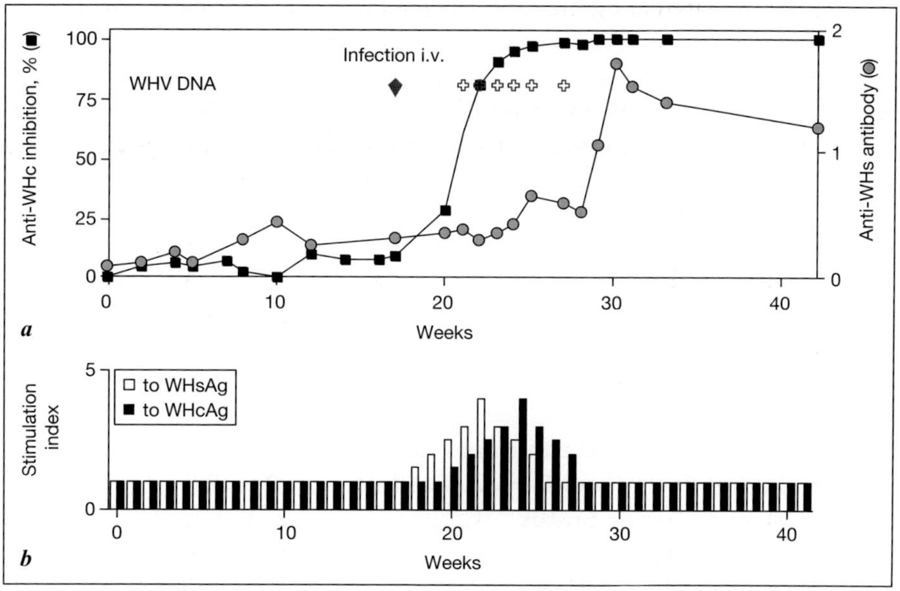

Fig. 3. Experimental infection of woodchucks. ***a*** Experimental infection of woodchucks is used to be initiated by intravenous injection of WHV. The WHV infection can be monitored by detection of WHV DNA using spot blot hybridization and detection of WHsAg using specific ELISA. Antibodies to WHcAg and WHsAg are detected by ELISAs. ***b*** The lymphoproliferative response to the WHV proteins is usually measurable during the viremic phase. The WHsAg-specific response appears early in the course of infection, while the response to WHcAg peaks later and is coincident with the appearance of anti-WHsAg.

the fact that outbred animals were used in these studies which might have had different alleles of MHC class II. Some peptides, on the other hand, like peptides 97–110 (100%), 110–119 (86%), 112–131 (55%) and 1–20 (53%), were recognized by the majority of woodchucks with acute self-limiting infection which strengthens previous findings which have shown that some immunodominant epitopes may be promiscuous. The importance of the immune response to epitope 97–110 has been demonstrated in subsequent experiments. Woodchucks immunized four times with this peptide showed a specific T-cell response and were protected from WHV infection, as no WHV DNA was detectable in serum and liver. We observed a specific and increasing T-cell response to peptide 97–110, and rWHcAg following immunization. The predominant T-cell response to WHV antigens during immunization and after challenge suggests that protection was primarily based on the cellular response (Th cells and/or CTLs). Likewise, immunization of mice with peptides derived from the nucleoprotein of lymphocytic choriomeningitis virus resulted in protection without detectable virus-neutralizing antibodies [42, 63]. Further experiments are needed to elucidate the mechanism of protection. Animals which developed chronic infection showed only a weak T-cell response. The majority of them were unable to recognize peptide 97–110 but developed T-cell response to other epitopes which are present at a low frequency in animals with acute resolving WHV infection. The appropriate immune response during the incubation period of WHV infection has to be considered as the critical period of virus-host interaction. Further studies are needed to characterize virus-specific CD8+ T cells in the woodchuck system in the peripheral blood and the liver to determine their contribution to elimination of virus replication and WHV-infected cells with cccDNA.

Failure of Appropriate Immune Response in the Incubation Period and Early Acute Infection Results in Chronic Carrier Status

Only weak or no T-helper responses are detected in chronic HBV/WHV carriers. The question arises whether the chronic outcome of hepadnaviral infection is related to failure to mount an early T-helper response or to loss of T cells during the acute phase.

Studies on the early immunological events following HBV infection in humans usually are limited due to the time interval between infection and onset of clinical symptoms. Only a very small number of patients could be tested so far [78]. As the majority of these cases represent self-limited courses, there are only few opportunities to examine the T-cell response in the acute phase associated with subsequent development of chronic HBV infection. The question whether chronic outcome is associated with an absent or suboptimal cellular immune response during the incubation period or early acute infection has been addressed in the woodchuck. WHV infection of neonate woodchucks led to development of a high carrier rate. The rate of chronic outcome depends on age at time of infection, viral strain and viral titer of inoculums. WHV strains W8 and W7 are closely related and differ from each other by few positions on their genomes [23]. They have identical precore and core proteins, identical small and middle surface proteins, and there are only 2 amino acid substitutions in each of the X protein and pre-S1 region of the envelope protein and 9 amino acid substitutions in the polymerase protein. Inoculation of neonatal woodchucks with W8 resulted in 11 resolved infections and 4 chronic carriers out of 15 infected woodchuck neonates [57]. In a second experiment, neonates were infected with W7, which consistently produces higher rates of chronicity. Inoculation of 19 neonatal woodchucks with W7 produced 19

grafts with HBV is a pertinent problem in liver transplantation, requiring the development of new treatment strategies. Living liver donation is a new option to optimize results of liver transplantation and may allow immune modulation of the donor prior to the operation. This was the reason to establish the technique of liver transplantation in the woodchuck, and to use adoptive transfer of the immune response to WHV from a donor to a WHV carrier woodchuck to prevent reinfection [12]. First we investigated reinfection with WHV. WHV-negative animals were selected as donors, whereas chronic carriers served as recipients for these experiments. Early after transplantation, membranous but no intracytoplasmic immunohistochemical staining for WHsAg was detected in the liver graft, which was negative for WHcAg as well as WHV DNA and RNA. WHV DNA replication intermediates and viral RNA were detected by Southern blot hybridization and Northern blot, respectively. The first sign of viral presence in the graft was WHsAg detected exclusively in the sinusoids. However, nearly all hepatocytes in the liver grafts of animals sacrificed at 3 and 10 weeks post-transplantation showed strong membranous (WHsAg) and intracytoplasmic (WHsAg and WHcAg) staining, which was higher in frequency and intensity than in carriers before transplantation. The apparently reduced level of WHV replication intermediates and viral RNA in the reinfected liver grafts compared with the carrier animals was caused by the severe morphological changes leading to a replacement of hepatocytes by extended portal infiltrates. The experimental liver transplantation proved that woodchuck represents a suitable model to study WHV reinfection after liver transplantation. The operative procedure was well tolerated. These promising results encouraged us to evaluate an adoptive immunotransfer by liver transplantation from immune animal to WHV carrier.

Animals negative for WHV were vaccinated using plasmids expressing WHsAg, WHcAg, and woodchuck IFN-γ in combination with a DNA vaccine [WHs antigen (WHsAg)] three times before liver donation. Chronic WHV carriers served as recipients. Control animals received the liver from non-immunized donors. The viral load in serum and liver tissue was monitored pre- and post-transplant for up to 11 weeks by dot blot, Northern blot, Southern blot, and immunohistochemistry for WHcAg and WHsAg.

Donor vaccination was effective, as indicated by the development of anti-WHc and anti-WHs antibodies [13]. Transplanting the livers of these donors resulted in a reduction of viral load in 2 of 3 animals. No viral DNA was detected in initial serum samples by dot-blot hybridization technique. However, polymerase chain reaction for viral DNA extracted from serum was always positive. Consistently, WHV replication intermediates and WHV RNA were absent in initial liver biopsies. Only few hepatocytes stained weakly positive for WHcAg and frequency, and the intensity of WHsAg-positive hepatocytes was low. However, reinfection that occurred with time through the WHV replication appeared to be limited as compared with controls. Liver transplantation from immunized donors to chronic carriers seems to be a promising strategy to reduce and delay severe reinfection, which may be applicable in a living liver transplantation program.

Conclusions

In recent years, the immune control of hepadnaviral infection has been studied intensively in animal models [24, 28, 74, 79]. Particularly the HBV-specific immune T-cell response was analyzed in the transgenic mouse model [25, 27]. In addition, immune transfer and immunization experiments in the mouse model provide interesting results, indicating the important role of antiviral cytokines IFN-γ and TNF-α as major mediators of the antiviral action of specific CTLs. Several findings in the animal models support the direct antiviral activity of cytokines: (1) In experimentally infected chimpanzees and woodchucks, a decline of replication of WHV/HBV has been observed prior to cell destruction as determined by elevated transaminases. (2) There is a direct correlation of intrahepatic expression of increased levels of IFN-γ and reduction of viral replication. (3) In the transgenic mouse model, antibodies to IFN-γ can completely abolish reduction of replication of HBV DNA. (4) Elimination of IFN-γ producing the specific CTLs by an anti-CD8 antibody is correlated to persistent replication until CD8+ cells reappear at later time points. These findings led to the hypothesis that cytokines suppress viral replication as a first step of viral clearance and on the other hand chronic HBV/WHV infection may be caused by a low expression of cytokines like IFN-γ. This hypothesis raised the question whether direct application or in vivo induction of cytokines could actually be used for the therapy of chronic HBV infection.

Our experiments in the woodchuck model with chronic virus infections revealed some aspects that have not yet been considered in the interpretations of the results from the transgenic mouse model.

It is not surprising that inflammatory cytokines including IFN-γ are expressed in liver tissues of chronically WHV-infected woodchucks. A number of IFN-stimulated genes were shown to be expressed in liver tissues. The expression of IFN-γ expressed in this context is, however, not sufficient to terminate WHV infection. It remains to be investigated whether the IFN-γ expression contributes at all to limit WHV replication during the chronic course of WHV infection.

The results about the therapeutic use of cytokine wIFN-γ in the woodchuck model are rather disappointing. wIFN-γ was applied on WHV-infected primary woodchuck hepatocytes but showed no significant antiviral effect even at cytotoxic concentrations [48]. Also, no significant suppression of WHV replication was achieved by in vivo application by adenoviral vector-mediated expression in liver [16]. Nevertheless, wIFN-γ has been clearly demonstrated to be biologically active in terms of induction of ISG expression in primary hepatocytes and in vivo. In addition, T cells from WHV carriers could not be stimulated by IL-12 to produce IFN-γ which is released by T cells of uninfected woodchucks [Fiedler et al., unpubl. results]. Taken together, with these findings the question arises whether an established WHV infection renders hepatocytes strongly resistant to wIFN-γ, indicating that chronic hepadnavirus infection is a result of viral resistance to cytokines or could be due to the changed cellular responsiveness to cytokines.

Thus, future investigations will take the major advantages of the woodchuck model as an authentic infection model. No other animal model is available that mimics the chronic course of hepadnaviral infection and presents the features in pathogenesis and virus-host interaction in such a satisfactory way as the woodchuck model.

References

1 Block TM, Lu X, Mehta AS, Blumberg BS, Tennant B, Ebling M, Korba B, Lansky DM, Jacob GS, Dwek RA: Treatment of chronic hepadnavirus infection in a woodchuck animal model with an inhibitor of protein folding and trafficking. Nat Med 1998;4:610–614.

2 Botta A, Lu M, Zhen X, Kemper T, Roggendorf M: Naturally occurring woodchuck hepatitis virus (WHV) deletion mutants in chronically WHV-infected woodchucks. Virology 2000;277:226–234.

3 Chen HS, Kaneko S, Girones R, Anderson RW, Hornbuckle WE, Tennant BC, Cote PJ, Gerin JL, Purcell RH, Miller RH: The woodchuck hepatitis virus X gene is important for establishment of virus infection in woodchucks. J Virol 1993;67:1218–1226.

4 Chen HS, Kew MC, Hornbuckle WE, Tennant BC, Cote PJ, Gerin JL, Purcell RH, Miller RH: The precore gene of the woodchuck hepatitis virus genome is not essential for viral replication in the natural host. J Virol 1992;66:5682–5684.

5 Cote PJ, Korba BE, Steinberg H, Ramirez-Mejia C, Baldwin B, Hornbuckle WE, Tennant BC, Gerin JL: Cyclosporin A modulates the course of woodchuck hepatitis virus infection and induces chronicity. J Immunol 1991;146:3138–3144.

6 Cote PJ, Korba BE, Baldwin B, Hornbuckle WE, Tennant BC, Gerin JL: Immunosuppression with cyclosporine during the incubation period of experimental woodchuck hepatitis virus infection increases the frequency of chronic infection in adult woodchucks. J Infect Dis 1992;166:628–631.

7 Cote PJ, Gerin JL: In vitro activation of woodchuck lymphocytes measured by radiopurine incorporation and interleukin-2 production: Implications for modeling immunity and therapy in hepatitis B virus infection. Hepatology 1995;22:687–699.

8 Cote PJ, Korba BE, Miller RH, Jacob JR, Baldwin BH, Hornbuckle WE, Purcell RH, Tennant BC, Gerin JL: Effects of age and viral determinants on chronicity as an outcome of experimental woodchuck hepatitis virus infection. Hepatology 2000;31:190–200.

9 Cote PJ, Toshkov I, Bellezza C, Ascenzi M, Roneker C, Ann Graham L, Baldwin BH, Gaye K, Nakamura I, Korba BE, Tennant BC, Gerin JL: Temporal pathogenesis of experimental neonatal

woodchuck hepatitis virus infection: Increased initial viral load and decreased severity of acute hepatitis during the development of chronic viral infection. Hepatology 2000;32:807–817.
10 Cullen JM, Li DH, Brown C, Eisenberg EJ, Cundy KC, Wolfe J, Toole J, Gibbs C: Antiviral efficacy and pharmacokinetics of oral adefovir dipivoxil in chronically woodchuck hepatitis virus-infected woodchucks. Antimicrob Agents Chemother 2001;45:2740–2745.
11 Cullen JM, Smith SL, Davis MG, Dunn SE, Botteron C, Cecchi A, Linsey D, Linzey D, Frick L, Paff MT, Goulding A, Biron K: In vivo antiviral activity and pharmacokinetics of (–)-*cis*-5-fluoro-1-[2-(hydroxymethyl)-1,3-oxathiolan-5-yl]cytosine in woodchuck hepatitis virus-infected woodchucks. Antimicrob Agents Chemother 1997;41:2076–2082.
12 Dahmen U, Li J, Dirsch O, Fiedler M, Lu M, Roggendorf M, Broelsch CE: A new model of hepatitis B virus reinfection: Liver transplantation in the woodchuck1. Transplantation 2002;74: 373–380.
13 Dahmen U, Dirsch O, Li J, Fiedler M, Lu M, Rispeter K, Picucci M, Broelsch CE, Roggendorf M: Adoptive transfer of immunity. A new strategy to interfere with severe hepatitis virus reinfection after woodchuck liver transplantation. Transplantation 2004;77:965–972.
14 Di Q, Summers J, Burch JB, Mason WS: Major differences between WHV and HBV in the regulation of transcription. Virology 1997;229:25–35.
15 Donello JE, Loeb JE, Hope TJ: Woodchuck hepatitis virus contains a tripartite posttranscriptional regulatory element. J Virol 1998;72:5085–5092.
16 Fiedler M, Rödicker F, Salucci V, Lu M, Aurisicchio L, Dahmen U, Li J, Dirsch O, Pützer BM, Palombo F, Roggendorf M: Helper-dependent adenoviral vector-mediated delivery of woodchuck specific genes for interferon alpha (IFN-α) and gamma (IFN-γ): IFN-α, but not IFN-γ reduces woodchuck hepatitis virus replication in chronic infection in vivo. J Virol 2004; 78:10111–10121.
17 Feitelson MA, Ranganathan PN, Clayton MM, Zhang SM: Partial characterization of the woodchuck tumor suppressor, p53, and its interaction with woodchuck hepatitis virus X antigen in hepatocarcinogenesis. Oncogene 1997;15:327–336.
18 Flajolet M, Tiollais P, Buendia MA, Fourel G: Woodchuck hepatitis virus enhancer I and enhancer II are both involved in N-myc2 activation in woodchuck liver tumors. J Virol 1998; 72:6175–6180.
19 Fourel G, Couturier J, Wei Y, Apiou F, Tiollais P, Buendia MA: Evidence for long range oncogene activation by hepadnavirus insertion. EMBO J 1994;13:2526–2534.
20 Galibert F, Chen TN, Mandard E: Localization and nucleotide sequence of the gene coding for the woodchuck hepatitis virus surface antigen: Comparison with the gene coding for the human hepatitis B virus surface antigen. Proc Natl Acad Sci USA 1981;78:5315–5319.
21 Garcia-Navarro R, Blanco-Urgoiti B, Berraondo P, Sanchez de la Rosa R, Vales A, Hervas-Stubbs S, Lasarte JJ, Borras F, Ruiz J, Prieto J: Protection against woodchuck hepatitis virus (WHV) infection by gene gun coimmunization with WHV core and interleukin-12. J Virol 2001; 75:9068–9076.
22 Genovesi EV, Lamb L, Medina I, Taylor D, Seifer M, Innaimo S, Colonno RJ, Clark JM: Antiviral efficacy of lobucavir (BMS-180194), a cyclobutyl-guanosine nucleoside analogue, in the woodchuck (*Marmota monax*) model of chronic hepatitis B virus infection. Antiviral Res 2000; 48:197–203.
23 Girones R, Cote PJ, Hornbuckle WE, Tennant BC, Gerin JL, Purcell RH, Miller RH: Complete nucleotide sequence of a molecular clone of woodchuck hepatitis virus that is infectious in the natural host. Proc Natl Acad Sci USA 1989;86:1846–1849.
24 Guidotti LG, Rochford R, Chung J, Shapiro M, Purcell R, Chisari FV: Viral clearance without destruction of infected cells during acute HBV infection. Science 1999;284:825–829.
25 Guidotti LG, Chisari FV: Noncytolytic control of viral infections by the innate and adaptive immune response. Annu Rev Immunol 2001;19:65–91.
26 Guidotti LG, Ando K, Hobbs MV, Ishikawa BT, Runkel L, Schreiber R, Chisari FV: Cytotoxic T lymphocytes inhibit hepatitis B virus gene expression by a noncytolytic mechanism in transgenic mice. Proc Natl Acad Sci USA 1994;91:3764–3768.
27 Guidotti LG, Ishkawa T, Hobbs MV, Matzke B, Schreiber R, Chisari FV: Intracellular inactivation of the hepatitis B virus by cytotoxic T lymphocytes. Immunity 1996;4:25–36.

28 Guo JT, Zhou H, Liu C, Alrich C, Saputelli J, Whitaker T, Inmaculada Barrasa M, Mason WS, Seeger C: Apoptosis and regeneration of hepatocytes during recovery from transient hepadnavirus infections. J Virol 2000;74:1495–1505.
29 Hervas-Stubbs S, Lasarte JJ, Sarobe P, Vivas I, Condreay L, Cullen JM, Prieto J, Borras-Cuesta F: T-helper cell response to woodchuck hepatitis virus antigens after therapeutic vaccination of chronically-infected animals treated with lamivudine. J Hepatol 2001;35:105–111.
30 Hodgson PD, Michalak TI: Augmented hepatic interferon-γ expression and T-cell influx characterize acute hepatitis progressing to recovery and residual lifelong virus persistence in experimental adult woodchuck hepatitis virus infection. Hepatology 2001;34:1049–1059.
31 Hodgson PD, Grant MD, Michalak TI: Perforin and Fas/Fas ligand-mediated cytotoxicity in acute and chronic woodchuck viral hepatitis. Clin Exp Immunol 1999;118:63–70.
32 Josephson L, Rutkowski JV, Paul K, Frigo T, Korba BE, Tennant B, Groman EV: Antiviral activity of a conjugate of adenine-9-β-*D*-arabinofuranoside 5′-monophosphate and a 9-kDa fragment of arabinogalactan. Antivir Ther 1996;1:147–156.
33 Kajino K, Jilbert AR, Saputelli J, Aldrich CE, Cullen J, Mason WS: Woodchuck hepatitis virus infections: Very rapid recovery after a prolonged viremia and infection of virtually every hepatocyte. J Virol 1994;68:5792–5803.
34 Klavinskis LS, Whitton JL, Joly E, Oldstone MBA: Vaccination and protection from a lethal viral infection, identification, incorporation, and use of cytotoxic T-lymphocyte glycoprotein epitope. Virology 1990;178:1213–1216.
35 Korba BE, Cote P, Hornbuckle W, Schinazi R, Gangemi JD, Tennant BC, Gerin JL: Enhanced antiviral benefit of combination therapy with lamivudine and interferon-α against WHV replication in chronic carrier woodchucks. Antivir Ther 2000;5:95–104.
36 Korba BE, Schinazi RF, Cote P, Tennant BC, Gerin JL: Effect of oral administration of emtricitabine on woodchuck hepatitis virus replication in chronically infected woodchucks. Antimicrob Agents Chemother 2000;44:1757–1760.
37 Korba BE, Cote P, Hornbuckle W, Tennant BC, Gerin JL: Treatment of chronic woodchuck hepatitis virus infection in the Eastern woodchuck (*Marmota monax*) with nucleoside analogues is predictive of therapy for chronic hepatitis B virus infection in humans. Hepatology 2000;31:1165–1175.
38 Kreuzfelder E, Menne S, Ferencic S, Roggendorf M, Grosse-Wilde H: Assessment of peripheral blood mononuclear cell proliferation by 2[^{3}H]adenine uptake in the woodchuck model. Clin Immunol Immunopathol 1996;78:223–227.
39 Lanford RE, Chavez D, Brasky KM, Burns RB, Ricco-Hesse R: Isolation of a hepadnavirus from the woolly monkey, a new world primate. Proc Natl Acad Sci USA 1998;95:5757–5761.
40 Le Guerhier F, Pichoud C, Jamard C, Guerret S, Chevallier M, Peyrol S, Hantz O, King I, Trepo C, Cheng YC, Zoulim F: Antiviral activity of β-*L*-2,3′-dideoxy-2′,3′-didehydro-5-fluorocytidine in woodchucks chronically infected with woodchuck hepatitis virus. Antimicrob Agents Chemother 2001;45:1065–1077.
41 Li DH, Havell EA, Brown CL, Cullen JM: Woodchuck lymphotoxin-α, -β and tumor necrosis factor genes: Structure, characterization and biological activity. Gene 2000;25:242, 295–305.
42 Li DH, Newbold JE, Cullen JM: Natural populations of woodchuck hepatitis virus contain variant precore and core sequences including a premature stop codon in the ε motif. Virology 1996; 220:256–262.
43 Lohrengel B, Lu M, Roggendorf M: Molecular cloning of the woodchuck cytokines: TNF-α, IFN-γ, and IL-6. Immunogenetics 1998;47:332–335.
44 Lohrengel B, Lu M, Roggendorf M: Expression and purification of woodchuck tumour necrosis factor-α. Cytokine 2000;12:573–577.
45 Lu M, Hilken G, Kruppenbacher J, Kemper T, Schirmbeck R, Reimann J, Roggendorf M: Immunization of woodchucks with plasmids expressing woodchuck hepatitis virus (WHV) core antigen and surface antigen suppresses WHV infection. J Virol 1999;73:281–289.
46 Lu M, Roggendorf M: Evaluation of new approaches to prophylactic and therapeutic vaccinations against hepatitis B viruses in the woodchuck model. Intervirology 2001;44:124–131.
47 Lu M, Hilken G, Yang D, Kemper T, Roggendorf M: Replication of naturally occurring woodchuck hepatitis virus deletion mutants in primary hepatocyte cultures and after transmission to naive woodchucks. J Virol 2002;75:3811–3818.

48 Lu M, Lohrengel B, Hilken G, Kemper T, Roggendorf M: Woodchuck interferon-γ upregulates major histocompatibility complex class I transcription but is unable to deplete woodchuck hepatitis virus replication intermediates and RNAs in persistently infected woodchuck primary hepatocytes. J Virol 2002;76:58–67.
49 Lu M, Klaes R, Menne S, Gerlich W, Stahl B, Dienes HP, Drebber U, Roggendorf M: Induction of antibodies to the PreS region of surface antigens of woodchuck hepatitis virus (WHV) in chronic carrier woodchucks by immunizations with WHV surface antigens. J Hepatol 2003; 39:405–413.
50 Maschke J, Menne S, Jacob JR, Kreuzfelder E, Tennant BC, Roggendorf M, Grosse-Wilde H: Thymidine utilization abnormality in proliferating lymphocytes and hepatocytes of the woodchuck. Vet Immunol Immunopathol 2001;6403:1–18.
51 Mason WS, Seal G, Summers J: Virus of Pekin ducks with structural and biological relatedness to human hepatitis B virus. J Virol 1980;36:829–836.
52 Mason WS, Cullen J, Moraleda G, Saputelli J, Aldrich CE, Miller DS, Tennant B, Frick L, Averett D, Condreay LD, Jilbert AR: Lamivudine therapy of WHV-infected woodchucks. Virology 1998;245:18–32.
53 Mason W, Litwin S: Pathogenesis of hepadnavirus infections; in Lai CL, Locarnini S (eds): Hepatitis B Virus. Human Virus Guides 1. London, International Medical Press, 2002, pp 99 ff.
54 Menne S, Maschke J, Tolle TK, Lu M, Roggendorf M: Characterization of T-cell response to woodchuck hepatitis virus core protein and protection of woodchucks from infection by immunization with peptides containing a T-cell epitope. J Virol 1997;71:65–74.
55 Menne S, Maschke J, Tolle T, Kreuzfelder E, Grosse-Wilde H, Roggendorf M: Determination of peripheral blood mononuclear cell responses to mitogens and woodchuck hepatitis virus core antigen in woodchucks by 5-bromo-2′-deoxyuridine or 2[^{3}H]adenine incorporation. Arch Virol 1997;142:511–521.
56 Menne S, Maschke J, Lu M, Grosse-Wilde H, Roggendorf M: T-cell response to woodchuck hepatitis virus (WHV) antigens during acute self-limited WHV infection and convalescence and after viral challenge. J Virol 1998;72:6083–6091.
57 Menne S, Roneker CA, Roggendorf M, Gerin JL, Cote PJ, Tennant BC: Deficiencies in the acute-phase cell-mediated immune response to viral antigens are associated with development of chronic woodchuck hepatitis virus infection following neonatal inoculation. J Virol 2002; 76:1769–1780.
58 Menne S, Roneker CA, Tennant BC, Korba BE, Gerin JL, Cote PJ: Immunogenic effects of woodchuck hepatitis virus surface antigen vaccine in combination with antiviral therapy: Breaking of humoral and cellular immune tolerance in chronic woodchuck hepatitis virus infection. Intervirology 2002;45:237–250.
59 Michalak TI, Hodgson PD, Churchill ND: Posttranscriptional inhibition of class I major histocompatibility complex presentation on hepatocytes and lymphoid cells in chronic woodchuck hepatitis virus infection. J Virol 2000;74:4483–4494.
60 Miller RH, Girones R, Cote PJ, Hornbuckle WE, Chestnut T, Baldwin BH, Korba BE, Tennant BC, Gerin JL, Purcell RH: Evidence against a requisite role for defective virus in the establishment of persistent hepadnavirus infections. Proc Natl Acad Sci USA 1990;87:9329–9332.
61 Nakamura I, Nupp JT, Cowlen M, Hall WC, Tennant BC, Casey JL, Gerin JL, Cote PJ: Pathogenesis of experimental neonatal woodchuck hepatitis virus infection: Chronicity as an outcome of infection is associated with a diminished acute hepatitis that is temporally deficient for the expression of interferon-γ and tumor necrosis factor-α messenger RNAs. Hepatology 2001; 33:439–447.
62 Nakamura I, Nupp JT, Rao BS, Buckler-White A, Engle RE, Casey JL, Gerin JL, Cote PJ: Cloning and characterization of partial cDNAs for woodchuck cytokines and CD3ε with applications for the detection of RNA expression in tissues by RT-PCR assay. J Med Virol 1997;53:85–95.
63 Oldstone MBA, Tishon A, Eddleston M, de la Torre JC, McKee T, Whitton JL: Vaccination to prevent persistent viral infection. J Virol 1993;67:4372–4378.
64 Peek SF, Cote PJ, Jacob JR, Toshkov IA, Hornbuckle WE, Baldwin BH, Wells FV, Chu CK, Gerin JL, Tennant BC, Korba BE: Antiviral activity of clevudine [*L*-FMAU, (1-(2-fluoro-5-methyl-β,*L*-arabinofuranosyl)uracil)] against woodchuck hepatitis virus replication and gene expression in chronically infected woodchucks (*Marmota monax*). Hepatology 2001;33: 254–266.

65 Pützer BM, Stiewe T, Rödicker F, Schildgen O, Rühm S, Dirsch O, Fiedler M, Dahmen U, Tennant B, Scherer C, Graham FL, Roggendorf M: Large nontransplanted hepatocellular carcinoma in woodchucks: Treatment with adenovirus-mediated delivery of interleukin-12/B7.1 genes. J Natl Cancer Inst 2001;93:472–479.
66 Roggendorf M, Tolle TK: The woodchuck: An animal model for hepatitis B virus infection in man. Intervirology 1995;38:100–112.
67 Salucci V, Lu M, Aurisicchio L, La Monica N, Roggendorf M, Palombo F: Expression of a new woodchuck IFN-α gene by a helper-dependent adenoviral vector in woodchuck hepatitis virus-infected primary hepatocytes. J Interferon Cytokine Res 2002;22:1027–1034.
68 Summers J, Smolec JM, Snyder R: A virus similar to human hepatitis B virus associated with hepatitis and hepatoma in woodchucks. Proc Natl Acad Sci USA 1978;75:4533–4537.
69 Summers J, Jilbert AR, Yang W, Aldrich CE, Saputelli J, Litwin S, Toll E, Mason WS: Hepatocyte turnover during resolution of a transient hepadnaviral infection. Proc Natl Acad Sci USA 2003; 100:11652–11659.
70 Tatti KM, Korba BE, Stang HL, Peek S, Gerin JL, Tennant BC, Schinazi RF: Mutations in the conserved woodchuck hepatitis virus polymerase FLLA and YMDD regions conferring resistance to lamivudine. Antiviral Res 2002;55:141–150.
71 Tennant BC: Woodchuck hepadnaviruses; in Zuckerman AJ, Thomas HC (eds): Viral Hepatitis: Scientific Basis and Clinical Management. London, Churchill Livingstone, 1997.
72 Tennant BC: Animal models of hepadnavirus-associated hepatocellular carcinoma. Clin Liver Dis 2001;5:43–68.
73 Tennant BC, Gerin JL: The woodchuck model of hepatitis B virus infection. ILAR J 2001;42: 89–102.
74 Thimme R, Wieland S, Steiger C, Ghrayeb J, Reimann KA, Purcell RH, Chisari F: CD8(+) T cells mediate viral clearance and disease pathogenesis during acute hepatitis B virus infection. J Virol 2003;77:68–76.
75 Wang Y, Menne S, Baldwin BH, Tennant BC, Gerin JL, Cote PJ: Kinetics of viremia and acute liver injury in relation to outcome of neonatal woodchuck hepatitis virus infection. J Med Virol 2004;72:406–415.
76 Wang Y, Menne S, Jacob JR, Tennant BC, Gerin JL, Cote PJ: Role of type 1 versus type 2 immune responses in liver during the onset of chronic woodchuck hepatitis virus infection. Hepatology 2003;37:771–780.
77 Warren KS, Heeney JL, Swan RA, Heriyanto S, Verschoor EJ: A new group of hepadnaviruses naturally infecting orangutans (*Pongo pygnaeus*). J Virol 1999;73:7860–7865.
78 Webster GJM, Reignat S, Maini MK, Whalley SA, Ogg GS, King A, Brown D, Amlot PL, Williams R, Vergani D, Dusheiko GM, Bertoletti A: Incubation phase of acute hepatitis B in man: Dynamic of cellular immune mechanisms. Hepatology 2000;32:1117–1124.
79 Wieland SF, Spangenberg HC, Thimme R, Purcell RH, Chisari FV: Expansion and contraction of the hepatitis B virus transcriptional template in infected chimpanzees. Proc Natl Acad Sci USA 2004;101:2129–2134.
80 Wu HL, Chen PJ, Lin HK, Lee RS, Lin HL, Liu CJ, Lee PJ, Lee JJ, Chen DS: Molecular cloning and expression of woodchuck granulocyte-macrophage colony stimulating factor. J Med Virol 2001;65:567–575.
81 Yamamoto T, Litwin S, Zhou T, Zhu Y, Condreay L, Furman P, Mason WS: Mutations of the woodchuck hepatitis virus polymerase gene that confer resistance to lamivudine and 2′-fluoro-5-methyl-β-*L*-arabinofuranosyluracil. J Virol 2002;76:1213–1223.
82 Yang DL, Lu M, Hou LJ, Roggenorf M: Molecular cloning and characterization of major histocompatibility complex class I cDNAs from woodchuck. Tissue antigens 2000;55:548–557.
83 Yang D, Roggendorf M, Lu M: Molecular characterization of CD28 and cytotoxic T-lymphocyte-associated antigen 4 (CTLA-4) of woodchuck (*Marmota monax*). Tissue Antigen 2003;62:225–232.
84 Zhang Z, Torii N, Hu Z, Jacob J, Liang TJ: X-deficient woodchuck hepatitis virus mutants behave like attenuated viruses and induce protective immunity in vivo. J Clin Invest 2001;108: 1523–1531.
85 Zhou T, Guo JT, Nunes FA, Molnar-Kimber KL, Wilson JM, Aldrich CE, Saputelli J, Litwin S, Condreay LD, Seeger C, Mason WS: Combination therapy with lamivudine and adenovirus causes

transient suppression of chronic woodchuck hepatitis virus infections. J Virol 2000;74: 11754–11763.

86 Zhou T, Saputelli J, Aldrich CE, Deslauriers M, Condreay LD, Mason WS: Emergence of drug-resistant populations of woodchuck hepatitis virus in woodchucks treated with the antiviral nucleoside lamivudine. Antimicrob Agents Chemother 1999;43:1947–1954.

87 Zhou JH, Ferencik S, Rebmann V, Yang DL, Lu M, Roggendorf M, Grosse-Wilde H: Molecular genetic and biochemical analysis of woodchuck (*Marmota monax*) MHC class I polymorphism. Tissue Antigen 2003;61:240–248.

88 Zhu Y, Cullen J, Aldrich CE, Saputelli J, Miller D, Seeger C, Mason WS, Jilbert AR: Adenovirus-based gene therapy during clevudine treatment of woodchucks chronically infected with woodchuck hepatitis virus. J Virol 2004 (submitted).

89 Zoulim F: Therapy of chronic hepatitis B virus infection: Inhibition of the viral polymerase and other antiviral strategies. Antiviral Res 1999;44:1–30.

90 Zoulim F, Le Guerhier F, Seignères B: Animal models for the study of HBV infection; in Lai CL, Locarnini S (eds): Hepatitis B Virus. Human Virus Guides 1. London, International Medical Press, 2002, pp 81 ff.

Prof. Dr. med. M. Roggendorf
Institute of Virology, University of Essen
Hufelandstrasse 55, DE–45122 Essen (Germany)
Tel. +49 201 723 3550, Fax +49 201 723 5929, E-Mail roggendorf@uni-essen.de

von Weizsäcker F, Roggendorf M (eds): Models of Viral Hepatitis.
Monogr Virol. Basel, Karger, 2005, vol 25, pp 25–32

Pathogenesis of Hepatitis B Virus in Transgenic Mice

Giovanni Sitia[a,b], *Matteo Iannacone*[a,c], *Francis V. Chisari*[a], *Luca G. Guidotti*[a]

[a]Department of Molecular and Experimental Medicine, The Scripps Research Institute, La Jolla, Calif., USA and Departments of [b]Infectious Diseases and [c]Internal Medicine, San Raffaele Scientific Institute, Milan, Italy

Hepatitis B virus (HBV) is a small, enveloped DNA virus that causes acute and chronic necroinflammatory liver disease and hepatocellular carcinoma [1]. HBV infection in immunocompetent adults usually results in transient liver disease and viral clearance. A small percentage of these patients (5–10%) develop chronic hepatitis associated with viral persistence. When neonates are infected, however, over 90% of them will become persistently infected, suffering different degrees of chronic liver disease. Unfortunately, cirrhosis and hepatocellular carcinoma are frequent complications of chronic HBV infection. Since HBV is not directly cytopathic for the hepatocyte, the immune response to viral antigens is thought to be responsible for both liver disease and viral clearance following HBV infection. Indeed, patients with acute viral hepatitis, who successfully clear the virus, mount a multispecific polyclonal CTL response to several HBV-encoded antigens [1]. In contrast, this response is absent or extremely weak in chronically infected patients who do not clear the virus [1, 2] and thus, it is believed that the outcome of HBV infection (viral clearance versus viral persistence) is determined primarily by the vigor and quality of the cellular immune response.

The experimental approaches to HBV pathogenesis have been difficult because the host range of HBV is limited to man and chimpanzees. Studies of HBV pathogenesis using models of HBV-related hepadnavirus infections in the woodchuck, ground squirrel and Pekin duck have also been difficult because the immune system of these outbred species has not been characterized.

Definitive analysis of the immunological mechanisms involved in HBV pathogenesis required the development of an inbred animal model with a well-defined immune system, i.e. the HBV transgenic mouse. In the course of those studies many other previously unknown aspects of HBV pathogenesis have been elucidated because of the unique power of the transgenic mouse system to replicate HBV in the primary hepatocyte in vivo.

Two lineages of transgenic mice containing complete copies of the HBV genome have been produced whose hepatocytes replicate the virus at high levels without any evidence of cytopathology [3]. These mice were generated by microinjection of a terminally redundant viral DNA construct 1.3 HBV genomes in length, containing only viral regulatory elements and no cellular promoters. Out of all four HBV RNAs produced in the liver of these animals, the two most abundant transcriptional products of the transgene (as occurs during natural infection) are the 3.5- and 2.1-kb RNA. The 3.5-kb RNA (or pregenomic) RNA is reverse transcribed by the viral polymerase into the HBV DNA replicative intermediates inside of viral nucleocapsid particles more abundant in centrilobular hepatocytes. As a consequence of efficient viral replication, ultrastructurally complete and infectious [4] viral particles that are morphologically indistinguishable from human-derived virions are detected at high levels in the transgenic mouse serum (between 107 and 108 viral particles per ml), further indicating that the HBV life cycle can be efficiently completed in the transgenic mouse hepatocyte [3].

Antiviral Mechanisms

The antiviral and immunopathological consequences of antigen recognition in this model were examined by administration of virus-specific CTLs. Surprisingly, the antiviral potential of the CTLs was shown to be primarily mediated by non-cytolytic mechanisms that involve the intrahepatic production of type 1 inflammatory cytokines by the CTLs [5–7]. These cytokines activate two functionally independent virocidal pathways: an early pathway that eliminates HBV nucleocapsid particles and their cargo of replicating viral genomes from the hepatocyte [8, 9]; and a later pathway that post-transcriptionally downregulates the viral RNA [10, 11]. In recent studies, it was shown that IFN-γ mediates most of the antiviral effect of the CTLs [12] and nitric oxide (NO) mediates most of the antiviral activity of IFN-γ [13].

One might predict from the foregoing that HBV-non-specific inflammatory responses of the liver could facilitate the clearance of HBV if they induce the local production of antiviral cytokines (such as IFN-γ and IFN-α/β) to which HBV is susceptible. Precisely these events have been shown to occur in the HBV transgenic mice during unrelated hepatotropic infections of the liver which include lymphocytic choriomeningitis virus (LCMV) [12, 14], adenovirus [12, 15], mouse cytomegalovirus (MCMV) [15], malaria [16] or *Schistosoma* [17] or after administration of recombinant murine IL-12 [18], a cytokine produced by antigen-presenting cells (APCs) that has the ability to induce IFN-γ secretion by T cells, natural killer (NK) and NKT cells. Along these lines, it was also shown that a single injection of α-galactosylceramide (α-GalCer), a glycolipid antigen presented to $V\alpha 14^+$, $NK1.1^+$ T cells by the non-classical MHC class I-like molecule CD1d, inhibits HBV replication by directly activating NKT cells to produce IFN-γ in the liver [19, 20]. Furthermore, HBV replication was inhibited in the transgenic animals by systemic administration of IFN-α [17], the IFN-α/β inducer poly-inosinic-polycytidylic acid complex (Poly-I/C) [9, 17] or IL18 [21]. Finally, recent studies have shown that an anti-CD40 agonistic mAb (αCD40) was sufficient to activate APCs within the liver and inhibit HBV replication non-cytopathically by a cytokine-dependent process [22].

Importantly, previous work has also produced evidence suggesting that non-cytopathic antiviral mechanisms may contribute to viral clearance during acute viral hepatitis in chimpanzees, thus validating the transgenic mouse studies in a natural infection model [4]. Moreover, cytokines known to abolish HBV replication from the hepatocyte also clear a persistent LCMV infection from the hepatocyte non-cytopathically, indicating that, like HBV, LCMV is also susceptible to intracellular inactivation by cytokine-induced antiviral mechanisms that are operative in the hepatocyte [23].

Absolute clearance requires elimination of the episomal covalently closed circular (CCC) HBV DNA species that serves during natural infection as the viral transcriptional template in the nucleus of the hepatocyte [24]. For unknown reasons, wild-type HBV transgenic mice do not produce CCC DNA, but they very efficiently express and replicate HBV using the integrated transgene as template [3]. It must be noted that low levels CCC DNA have been found in the liver of these same HBV transgenic mice once they were crossed with hepatocyte nuclear factor 1α-null mice [25]. This suggests that the impairment on CCC DNA synthesis in the mouse hepatocyte is not absolute. The absent or very low levels of CCC DNA detected in the transgenic mice, however, do not allow to know whether this viral species is also susceptible to cytokine-mediated control in this model. Nonetheless, since CCC DNA is abolished in the chimp infection model in the absence of massive destruction or regeneration of hepatocytes and in the presence of inflammatory cytokines [4], it is possible that cytokine-dependent pathways may contribute to the elimination of CCC DNA from the resting hepatocyte as well.

Immunopathological Mechanisms

Liver disease in the CTL transfer model begins with antigen recognition by the CTLs and delivery of signals that trigger the death of the hepatocyte by apoptosis [26]. Following antigen recognition, the CTL become activated and recruit many host-derived inflammatory cells into the liver, thereby contributing to the formation of necroinflammatory foci in which apoptotic hepatocytes and CTL are outnumbered by host-derived lymphomononuclear (such as lymphocytes, NK cells and macrophages) and polymorphonuclear (such as neutrophils and eosinophils) inflammatory cells [27, 28]. These necroinflammatory foci are scattered throughout the liver parenchyma and cause a focal lesion histologically identical to classical viral hepatitis in man.

Recruitment of host-derived antigen non-specific inflammatory cells into the liver is a process that is associated with the intrahepatic production of chemokines and it is likely to contribute to the pathogenesis of liver disease. Indeed, a recent study showed that blocking the chemokines CXCL9 and CXCL10 reduces the intrahepatic recruitment of host-derived lymphomononuclear cells and the severity of liver disease [28]. In that study it was also shown that CXCL9 and CXCL10 are rapidly and strongly induced in the liver after CTL transfer and the transferred CTL produce neither chemokine; rather, they activate (via the secretion of IFN-γ) hepatocytes and non-parenchymal cells of the liver to produce them [28].

The association of reduced liver disease with reduced recruitment of antigen non-specific lymphomononuclear cells implies that these cells can amplify the liver damage initiated by the antigen-specific CTLs. Similar mechanisms may contribute to the pathogenesis of viral hepatitis in man, where, like in our system, the number of HBV-specific T cells detected in the liver is outnumbered by recruited non-virus-specific T cells [2, 29] and other inflammatory cells [30]. The pathogenetic mechanisms whereby antigen-non-specific lymphomononuclear cells may induce liver damage are not understood. Future studies will attempt to address this important issue.

We recently showed that depletion of Gr-1$^+$ cells also reduces the severity of liver disease in this model. Gr-1$^+$ cells include polymorphonuclear neutrophils (PMNs) [31], plasmacytoid dendritic cells (pDCs) [32–34] and a subset of monocytes/macrophages [35–37]. Interestingly, depletion of Gr-1$^+$ cells completely blocks the recruitment of all Gr-1$^-$ intrahepatic lymphomononuclear into the liver despite the fact that many chemokines (including CXCL9 and CXCL10) are induced at high levels in the organ [38]. These results indicate that Gr-1$^+$ cells are necessary for the intrahepatic recruitment of antigen non-specific Gr-1$^-$ lymphomononuclear cells and they suggest that functions by Gr-1^+ cells in addition to chemokine induction are necessary for the recruitment process to occur.

These functions may include the release of the matrix-degrading metalloproteinases (MMPs) by PMNs or other Gr-1^+ cells. While it is not known whether pDCs or Gr-1^+ monocytes/macrophages produce MMPs, PMNs are known to produce high levels of collagenases (such as MMP-8, neutrophil collagenase) and gelatinases (such as MMP-9, gelatinase B) [39]. The major action of these enzymes involves the remodeling of the extracellular matrix, a process that is thought to facilitate leukocyte trafficking through endothelial barriers and solid organs [39].

In keeping with this, in preliminary studies we showed that following CTL transfer various MMPs are rapidly induced in the liver. Interestingly, MMP-8 and MMP-9 (known to be produced by PMNs [39]) are not induced in anti-Gr-1-treated mice, while MMP-2, MMP-3, MMP-7, MMP-12, MMP-13 and MMP-14 (known to be produced by many other myeloid and non-myeloid cell types [39]) are induced, suggesting that Gr-1^+ cells, especially PMNs, are the likely source of MMP-8 and MMP-9 in our system. Since depletion of Gr-1^+ cells also inhibits CTL-induced recruitment of antigen-non-specific inflammatory cells into the liver [38], the tight association between MMP-8 and MMP-9 activities and IHL recruitment is compatible with the hypothesis that these enzymes facilitate leukocyte trafficking through the endothelial barrier and entry into the liver parenchyma.

To test this hypothesis, we inhibited MMP activity in vivo (via the hydrodynamic injection of a plasmid encoding the tissue inhibitor of matrix metalloproteinases TIMP-1) and we monitored whether this altered the intrahepatic recruitment and pathogenetic effector functions of HBV-specific CTLs and other inflammatory cells in our system (fig. 1). The enhanced expression of TIMP-1 inhibited the induction of MMP activity and reduced the CTL-induced recruitment of host-derived lymphomononuclear cells into the liver and the attending liver disease, indicating that the recruitment of these cells requires MMP activity. The data is compatible with the hypothesis that PMNs represent the first cell type to be recruited into the liver following antigen recognition by the CTLs. According to this hypothesis, the production of MMPs by PMNs could remodel the extracellular matrix and facilitate the trafficking of lymphomononuclear cells through the endothelial barrier and into the liver parenchyma in response to their own chemoattractants.

In conclusion, the production of transgenic mice has created the opportunity to examine several aspects of HBV pathogenesis that could not be approached in any other experimental system. Undoubtedly, the transgenic mouse model will help us to answer many more questions that still remain.

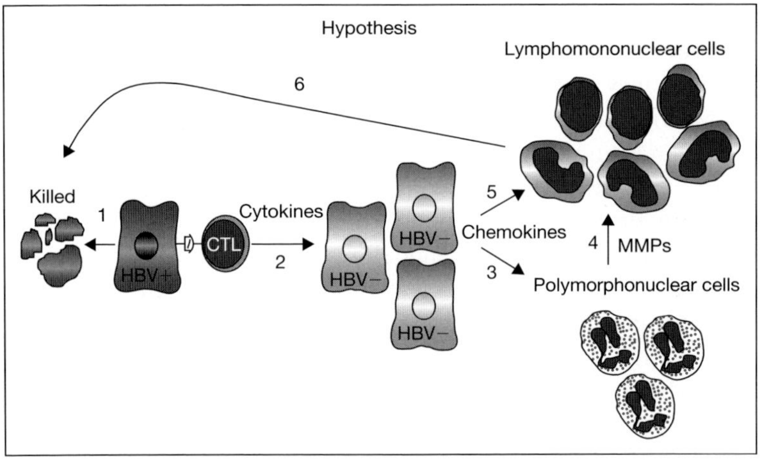

Fig. 1. Role of antigen-specific and non-specific inflammatory cells in the pathogenesis of HBV: *Hypothesis*. After antigen recognition, HBV-specific CTL kill a small number of hepatocytes (1), and produce antiviral cytokines (2) that inhibit HBV replication noncytopathically in a greater number of cells. The same cytokines can activate parenchymal and non-parenchymal cells of the liver to produce chemokines (3) that recruit antigen non-specific polymorphonuclear cells (i.e. neutrophils) into the organ. Production of MMPs by these cells (4) in addition to chemokine induction (5) may contribute to the migration of antigen non-specific lymphomononuclear cells (i.e. NK cells, T cells and macrophages) into the liver and the amplification of the liver disease initiated by the CTL (6).

Acknowledgements

We are indebted to Drs. Stefan Wieland, Kazuki Ando, Tetsuya Ishikawa, Kazuhiro Kakimi, Masanori Isogawa, Yasunari Nakamoto, Kiminori Kimura, Lisa Tsui, Victoria Cavanaugh, Valerie Pasquetto, Monte Hobbs, Rosemary Rochford, Iain Campbell, Persephone Borrow and Michael Oldstone who have contributed to the studies described in this paper. We are also grateful to Drs. Laura Runkel and Heinz Schaller for their active collaboration in the production of HBV transgenic mice. Finally, we want to thank Jenny Price for embryo microinjection, Patricia Fowler, Brent Matzke, Heike Mendez, Rick Koch, Sadie Medrano and Margie Chadwell for outstanding technical assistance. This work was supported by grants CA40489 (F.V.C.) and AI40696 (L.G.G.) from the National Institutes of Health. This is manuscript No. 16200-MEM from the Scripps Research Institute.

References

1 Chisari FV, Ferrari C: Hepatitis B virus immunopathogenesis. Annu Rev Immunol 1995;13:29–60.
2 Maini MK, Boni C, Lee CK, et al: The role of virus-specific CD8(+) cells in liver damage and viral control during persistent hepatitis B virus infection. J Exp Med 2000;191:1269–1280.

3 Guidotti LG, Matzke B, Schaller H, Chisari FV: High-level hepatitis B virus replication in transgenic mice. J Virol 1995;69:6158–6169.
4 Guidotti LG, Rochford R, Chung J, Shapiro M, Purcell R, Chisari FV: Viral clearance without destruction of infected cells during acute HBV infection. Science 1999;284:825–829.
5 Guidotti LG, Chisari FV: Cytokine-induced viral purging–role in viral pathogenesis. Curr Opin Microbiol 1999;2:388–391.
6 Guidotti LG, Chisari FV: Cytokine-mediated control of viral infections. Virology 2000; 273:221–227.
7 Guidotti LG, Chisari FV: Noncytolytic control of viral infections by the innate and adaptive immune response. Annu Rev Immunol 2001;19:65–91.
8 Guidotti LG, Ishikawa T, Hobbs MV, Matzke B, Schreiber R, Chisari FV: Intracellular inactivation of the hepatitis B virus by cytotoxic T lymphocytes. Immunity 1996;4:25–36.
9 Wieland SF, Guidotti LG, Chisari FV: Intrahepatic induction of alpha/beta interferon eliminates viral RNA-containing capsids in hepatitis B virus transgenic mice. J Virol 2000;74:4165–4173.
10 Tsui LV, Guidotti LG, Ishikawa T, Chisari FV: Post-transcriptional clearance of hepatitis B virus RNA by cytotoxic T lymphocyte-activated hepatocytes. Proc Natl Acad Sci USA 1995;92: 12398–12402.
11 Heise T, Guidotti LG, Cavanaugh VJ, Chisari FV: Hepatitis B virus RNA-binding proteins associated with cytokine-induced clearance of viral RNA from the liver of transgenic mice. J Virol 1999;73:474–481.
12 McClary H, Koch R, Chisari FV, Guidotti LG: Relative sensitivity of hepatitis B virus and other hepatotropic viruses to the antiviral effects of cytokines. J Virol 2000;74:2255–2264.
13 Guidotti LG, McClary H, Loudis JM, Chisari FV: Nitric oxide inhibits hepatitis B virus replication in the livers of transgenic mice. J Exp Med 2000;191:1247–1252.
14 Guidotti LG, Borrow P, Hobbs MV, et al: Viral cross talk: Intracellular inactivation of the hepatitis B virus during an unrelated viral infection of the liver. Proc Natl Acad Sci USA 1996;93: 4589–4594.
15 Cavanaugh VJ, Guidotti LG, Chisari FV: Inhibition of hepatitis B virus replication during adenovirus and cytomegalovirus infections in transgenic mice. J Virol 1998;72:2630–2637.
16 Pasquetto V, Guidotti LG, Kakimi K, Tsuji M, Chisari FV: Host-virus interactions during malaria infection in hepatitis B virus transgenic mice. J Exp Med 2000;192:529–536.
17 McClary H, Koch R, Chisari FV, Guidotti LG: Inhibition of hepatitis B virus replication during *Schistosoma mansoni* infection in transgenic mice. J Exp Med 2000;192:289–294.
18 Cavanaugh VJ, Guidotti LG, Chisari FV: Interleukin-12 inhibits hepatitis B virus replication in transgenic mice. J Virol 1997;71:3236–3243.
19 Kakimi K, Guidotti LG, Koezuka Y, Chisari FV: Natural killer T cell activation inhibits hepatitis B virus replication in vivo. J Exp Med 2000;192:921–930.
20 Kakimi K, Lane TE, Chisari FV, Guidotti LG: Cutting edge: Inhibition of hepatitis B virus replication by activated NK T cells does not require inflammatory cell recruitment to the liver. J Immunol 2001;167:6701–6705.
21 Kimura K, Kakimi K, Wieland S, Guidotti LG, Chisari FV: Interleukin-18 inhibits hepatitis B virus replication in the livers of transgenic mice. J Virol 2002;76:10702–10707.
22 Kimura K, Kakimi K, Wieland S, Guidotti LG, Chisari FV: Activated intrahepatic antigen-presenting cells inhibit hepatitis B virus replication in the liver of transgenic mice. J Immunol 2002;169: 5188–5195.
23 Guidotti LG, Borrow P, Brown A, McClary H, Koch R, Chisari FV: Noncytopathic clearance of lymphocytic choriomeningitis virus from the hepatocyte. J Exp Med 1999;189:1555–1564.
24 Summers J: The replication cycle of hepatitis B viruses. Cancer 1988;61:1957–1962.
25 Raney AK, Eggers CM, Kline EF, et al: Nuclear covalently closed circular viral genomic DNA in the liver of hepatocyte nuclear factor 1α-null hepatitis B virus transgenic mice. J Virol 2001; 75:2900–2911.
26 Ando K, Guidotti LG, Wirth S, et al: Class I-restricted cytotoxic T lymphocytes are directly cytopathic for their target cells in vivo. J Immunol 1994;152:3245–3253.
27 Ando K, Moriyama T, Guidotti LG, et al: Mechanisms of class I restricted immunopathology. A transgenic mouse model of fulminant hepatitis. J Exp Med 1993;178:1541–1554.

28 Kakimi K, Lane TE, Wieland S, et al: Blocking chemokine responsive to γ2-interferon (IFN)-γ inducible protein and monokine induced by IFN-γ activity in vivo reduces the pathogenetic but not the antiviral potential of hepatitis B virus-specific cytotoxic T lymphocytes. J Exp Med 2001;194:1755–1766.
29 Bertoletti A, Maini MK: Protection or damage: A dual role for the virus-specific cytotoxic T lymphocyte response in hepatitis B and C infection? Curr Opin Immunol 2000;12:403–408.
30 Ishak KG: Light microscopic morphology of viral hepatitis. Am J Clin Pathol 1976;65:787–827.
31 Lagasse E, Weissman IL: Flow cytometric identification of murine neutrophils and monocytes. J Immunol Methods 1996;197:139–150.
32 Nakano H, Yanagita M, Gunn MD: CD11c(+)B220(+)Gr-1(+) cells in mouse lymph nodes and spleen display characteristics of plasmacytoid dendritic cells. J Exp Med 2001;194:1171–1178.
33 Asselin-Paturel C, Boonstra A, Dalod M, et al: Mouse type I IFN-producing cells are immature APCs with plasmacytoid morphology. Nat Immunol 2001;2:1144–1150.
34 Dalod M, Hamilton T, Salomon R, et al: Dendritic cell responses to early murine cytomegalovirus infection: Subset functional specialization and differential regulation by interferon α/β. J Exp Med 2003;197:885–898.
35 Bronte V, Apolloni E, Cabrelle A, et al: Identification of a CD11b(+)/Gr-1(+)/CD31(+) myeloid progenitor capable of activating or suppressing CD8(+) T cells. Blood 2000;96:3838–3846.
36 Henderson RB, Hobbs JA, Mathies M, Hogg N: Rapid recruitment of inflammatory monocytes is independent of neutrophil migration. Blood 2003;102:328–335.
37 Mordue DG, Sibley LD: A novel population of Gr-1^{+}-activated macrophages induced during acute toxoplasmosis. J Leukoc Biol 2003;74:1015–1025.
38 Sitia G, Isogawa M, Kakimi K, Wieland SF, Chisari FV, Guidotti LG: Depletion of neutrophils blocks the recruitment of antigen-nonspecific cells into the liver without affecting the antiviral activity of hepatitis B virus-specific cytotoxic T lymphocytes. Proc Natl Acad Sci USA 2002;99:13717–13722.
39 Sternlicht MD, Werb Z: How matrix metalloproteinases regulate cell behavior. Annu Rev Cell Dev Biol 2001;17:463–516.

Luca G. Guidotti
The Scripps Research Institute, Department of Molecular and Experimental Medicine
10550 North Torrey Pines Road, La Jolla, CA 92037 (USA)
Tel. +1 858 7842758, Fax +1 858 7842960, E-Mail guidotti@scripps.edu

von Weizsäcker F, Roggendorf M (eds): Models of Viral Hepatitis.
Monogr Virol. Basel, Karger, 2005, vol 25, pp 33–41

Transfer of HBV Genomes into Mice

Heike Oberwinkler[a], *Andreas Untergasser*[a], *Martin Sprinzl*[b], *Ulrike Protzer*[a]

[a]Molecular Infectiology at the Center for Molecular Medicine Cologne, Institute for Medical Microbiology, Immunology and Hygiene, University of Cologne, Cologne, and [b]First Medical Department, University Hospital Mainz, Mainz, Germany

Chronic hepatitis B is one of the most common and most severe human infectious diseases worldwide. Currently, 5% of the world's population are persistently infected with hepatitis B virus (HBV) [1]. Infected individuals are at high risk of developing liver cirrhosis and, eventually, hepatocellular carcinoma. While an effective vaccine is available, current treatment regimens for hepatitis B are costly and often have limiting side effects [2, 3].

The causative agent of the disease is human HBV, the prototype member of the family of hepadnaviridae. These small, DNA-containing viruses replicate through reverse transcription but, in contrast to retroviruses, do not integrate into the host cell genome for replication [4]. Infectious virions have a lipoprotein envelope with large (L), medium (M) and small (S) envelope proteins and contain a nucleocapsid. This harbors a small (3–3.2 kb), partially double-stranded relaxed circular DNA (rcDNA) genome with the viral replication enzyme, P protein, covalently attached. After entry into the host cell, the genome is delivered to the nucleus and transformed into covalently closed circular DNA (cccDNA) that serves as a template for transcription. All genomic and subgenomic transcripts are translated into protein. The messenger RNA (mRNA) for the core and the P protein serves, in addition, as an RNA pregenome. It is co-packaged with P protein into newly forming capsids where it is reverse transcribed by the enzyme into DNA [for reviews, see 5, 6] (fig. 1).

One characteristic property of the hepadnaviruses is their high species and tissue specificity: HBV infects only humans and humanoid primates. It is not infectious for laboratory animals, which are genetically and immunologically well defined because they lack specific receptors. HBV only replicates in

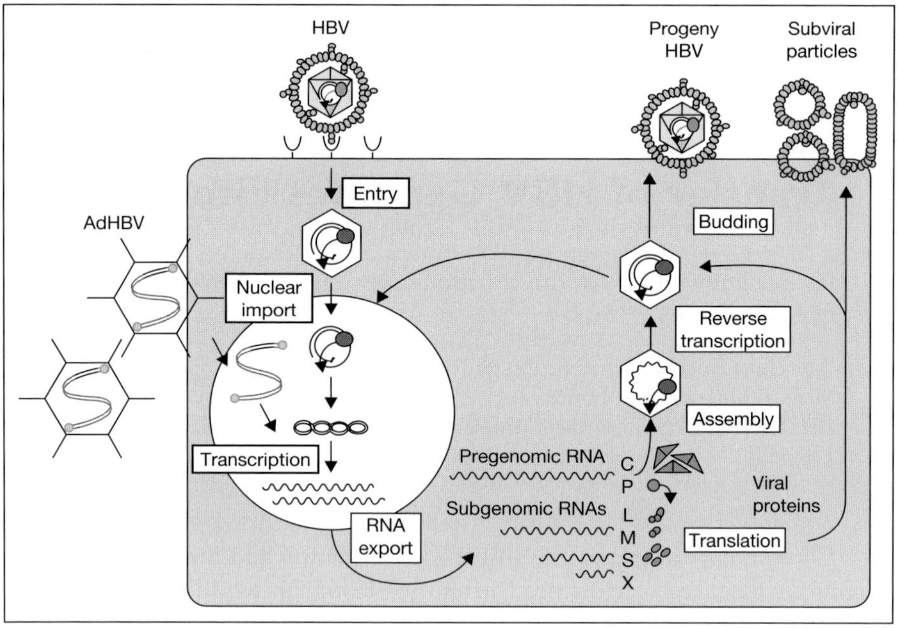

Fig. 1. Adenovirus-mediated transfer of HBV genomes into cells. Adenoviral vectors (AdHBV) containing replication-competent 1.3-fold HBV genomes allow to bypass the natural, receptor-mediated uptake of HBV. In permissive hepatocytes, AdHBV initiates the full HBV replication cycle (for details see text), whereby the recombinant AdHBV-genome instead of HBV cccDNA serves as the initial transcription template. By nuclear import of newly formed HBV capsids, however, cccDNA is established if the cellular machinery allows the nuclear import.

hepatocytes in its natural genome context. Besides virus uptake, viral promoters and enhancers confer hepatocyte specificity during replication [5, 7].

The development of new treatment strategies remains a major goal but is hindered by the lack of cell lines or a small animal model infectable with HBV that would allow testing. All HBVs are characterized by their high species and tissue specificity. Only primary human or primate hepatocytes are fully permissive for HBV, and chimpanzees are the only animals that can be infected with HBV. Consequently, only one permissive cell line [8] and no convenient small animal model is available that allows to study HBV infection.

HBV-transgenic mice [9] were generated which proved to be very useful for immunological studies and to study the control of HBV replication by the host immune system. Using that model, tremendous advance in our understanding of HBV-host interaction has been achieved [10]. However, transgenic mice do neither allow studying the onset, nor the establishment of HBV infection or viral dynamics during acute infection. As transgenic animals, these mice do not raise an immune response against HBV or its gene products. Furthermore, HBV replicates – unlike in natural infection – from an integrated genome, which cannot be eliminated.

Therefore, alternative small animal models were developed in which HBV genomes are introduced into hepatocytes by different means. These models enable us to study aspects of the establishment of HBV infection and of the immune response during acute infection, to compare the replication capacity of mutant viruses and to test prevention strategies.

Initially, direct injection of naked DNA into the livers of mice or rats was employed [11–13], but only a minor part of the hepatocytes was reached. Since in mice and rats the virus cannot spread, this led only to a very low level of replication. In mice and rats, a high number of hepatocytes must initially be targeted to achieve an easily detectable replication level. Thus, more efficient transfer systems were developed. One system employs adenoviral vectors for that purpose [14] (fig. 1), the other system takes advantage of the fact that DNA is preferentially taken up by hepatocytes when injected in a large volume of fluid [15]. Both systems allow to efficiently initiate HBV replication across the species barrier in the livers of a broad range of animals because they circumvent receptor-mediated uptake of HBV particles. We will discuss the adenovirus-mediated transfer of HBV genomes, which was developed in our laboratory, and will then compare it to other available animal models of HBV infection.

HBV Genome Transfer using Adenoviral Vectors

The adenovirus-mediated genome transfer efficiently initiates hepadnavirus replication in established cell lines, in primary hepatocytes from various species [14, 16] and in the livers of mice [14, 17]. Adenoviral vectors transfer 1.3-fold HBV genomes (AdHBV) from which infectious HBV is produced at high titers and with high liver specificity. These HBV constructs had proven superior over other replication-competent HBV constructs in transgenic mice [9] and were used for a baculovirus-mediated HBV genome transfer [18].

Following adenoviral genome transfer, HBV starts to replicate using the extra-chromosomal AdHBV genome as a transcription template. From day 2 after transduction, HBV proteins, genomic RNA and replicative DNA intermediates were detected [14]. Detection of covalently closed circular DNA in hepatoma cell lines and in primary hepatocytes indicated that an intracellular replication cycle independent from the transferred linear viral genome was established [14, 16]. Infectious hepatitis B virions were released into the culture medium of hepatoma cells or primary hepatocytes and into the serum of mice following AdHBV transduction [14, 17].

Adenoviral vectors became our first choice to transfer HBV genomes in order to establish an HBV replication system. Firstly, a broad range of immortalized and primary cells can be transduced using adenoviral vectors and the amount of transduced DNA can be controlled by varying the dose of recombinant adenovirus [19]. Secondly, of all known gene delivery vectors, adenoviral vectors most efficiently transfer foreign DNA into the livers of a broad variety of experimental animals [20, 21]. In the liver, they predominantly infect hepatocytes [22] – the site of HBV replication in natural infection. Thirdly, using adenoviral vectors, hepadnaviral replication is initiated from an extrachromosomal template as in natural infection.

In parallel to AdHBV, recombinant HBV-baculoviruses have been developed. They successfully initiated HBV replication in HepG2 hepatoma cells and lead to the establishment of a cccDNA pool in these cells [18]. There are, however, distinct disadvantages of baculovirus vectors. So far, baculoviruses were only shown to deliver HBV genomes into HepG2 cells [18, 23]. Neither mouse nor human primary hepatocytes are transduced at a sufficient number [pers. unpubl. observation]. Baculoviruses enter mammalian liver cells by an unspecific endosomal rather than by receptor-mediated uptake [24, 25]. Therefore, they transduce multiple DNA copies into few susceptible cells [24]. In addition, baculovirus-mediated gene transfer is restricted to certain species [24] and – most importantly – conventional baculovirus vectors are not suitable for gene transfer into experimental animals in vivo because they are rapidly inactivated by the complement system [26].

Commonly used adenoviral vectors are derived from a modified human adenovirus serotype 5. First-generation vector genomes include the entire adenoviral DNA sequence except of genes responsible for the initiation and propagation of adenoviral replication. This region is named E1 in respect to their early expression during the adenoviral replication cycle and was replaced by the HBV genome construct. Additional deletions in region E3 reduce adenoviral genome size and facilitate integration of transgenes without exceeding the adenoviral encapsidation capacity [27]. Detailed technical information about the generation of such adenoviral vectors for an HBV genome transfer is given in Sprinzl et al. [17].

The mouse probably is the most useful animal for the experimental analysis of various molecular and clinical aspects of HBV infection, because mice are easy to breed and to keep and many genetic variants are available. The mouse genome has been sequenced and the immune system is well characterized. AdHBV allows to initiate HBV replication in mice easily and reproducibly following intravenous injection [14, 17]. AdHBV-infected mice will allow studying the immune response against HBV in more detail, comparing viral mutants for their replication competence and pathogenicity, and testing of new prevention strategies. Establishment of long-term virus replication and repeated infection with an AdHBV vector, however, are limited by the host immune response towards the adenoviral vectors [30, 31]. In addition, effects of adenoviral vectors on cell metabolism and cell growth and their cytotoxicity limit the application of the recombinant AdHBV.

The adenoviral transfer of HBV genomes into adult mice does mimic an acute HBV infection. HBeAg and HBsAg secretion starts 1–2 days after AdHBV infection remains constant for 10–14 days and thereafter slowly declines. HBV viremia is maximal from day 3 to day 6 and remains detectable up to day 21 [A. Untergasser and U. Protzer, in preparation]. HBV-specific T cell response starts at day 7 [K. Kakimi and F. Chisari, submitted]. At days 24–34, in most animals HBsAg has disappeared from the peripheral blood and anti-HBs antibodies become detectable. With AdHBV, not only adult, but also neonatal animals can be infected resulting in long-term HBV replication. Thus, AdHBV allows to mimic acute infection in adult mice and vertical transmission in neonatal mice [pers. unpubl. results].

Because of the high immunogenicity and an apparent toxicity of first-generation adenoviral vectors, so called 'gutless', 'high-capacity' or 'helper dependent' adenoviral vectors (HDAd) have been developed which are devoid of all adenoviral coding sequences [32]. They are better tolerated than the first-generation vectors and allow persistent gene expression [33, 34]. Therefore, the construction of HDAdHBV is currently under way.

Alternative Models of HBV Infection

In the absence of suitable in vitro or in vivo infection systems for HBV, different experimental models are in use to study HBV infection. Two related animal viruses are used in their natural hosts: the duck HBV (DHBV; [35]), which infects Peking ducks, and the woodchuck HBV [36]. However, avian and mammalian hepadnaviruses differ in genome structure [35] and even between the closely related mammalian viruses – WHV and HBV – differences exist, e.g. in transcriptional regulation [37]. A tree shrew species, *Tupaia belangeri*, was reported to be susceptible to HBV infection [38, 39], but apparently carries the virus only transiently. Infection studies in all these models are limited by the fact that Peking ducks, woodchucks and tupaias genetically are badly characterized and that only few tools are available to study the immune response.

Recent developments therefore focus on mice. These developments include immunodeficient mice in which stably transfected HBV-producing immortalized liver cells are implanted [40], or human hepatocytes are engrafted [29]. Alternatively, B- and T-cell-deficient mice were used whose livers are repopulated with xenogenic hepatocytes [28, 41]. In the latter two models, the implanted human hepatocytes can be infected with HBV. Although these models seem very attractive because they represent an HBV infection model in the mouse, their availability is very limited due to the limited availability of human hepatocytes. Furthermore, to set up these models is very laborious, and they utilize immunodeficient animals unable to raise an immune response against the virus.

An alternative used early on was direct injection or cationic lipid-mediated transfer of naked viral DNA into the livers of animals [11–13, 42, 43]. By that way, however, the naked DNA only reached a small proportion of the hepatocytes and HBV replication was barely detectable [11]. To increase the efficacy of the DNA transfer, Yang et al. [15] used the hydrodynamic injection technique. This technique was originally described by Liu et al. [44] as a hydrodynamics-based transfection for expressing transgenes in mice. The fast injection of plasmid DNA in a high volume (1.6 ml in an 18- to 20-gram mouse) into the tail vein resulted in high level gene expression in the liver and low level gene expression in kidney, spleen, heart and lung [44]. Expression levels peaked 8 h post-injection and decreased to 1/1,000 of the original level by day 6 post-injection [44].

The advantage of the hydrodynamic injection of HBV-DNA is that only plasmid DNA is needed and no production of adenoviral vectors is necessary. This makes it easier for example to test large series of HBV variants. Biosafety concerns, which may be raised when adenoviral vectors are used, do not apply for plasmid DNA. Furthermore, studies on the immune response against HBV are not affected by an overlying anti-adeno immune response.

The disadvantage of the hydrodynamic injection is that it is mainly restricted to adult animals. It does not allow to infect neonatal animals as the adenoviral genome transfer does. Furthermore, hydrodynamic injection causes significant damage in the liver and irritation of the animals by the injection of large volumes of fluid. Hydrodynamic injection causes a transient irregularity of the heart function and a sharp increase in venous pressure resulting in retrograde perfusion of the liver [45]. In the liver, fenestrae in liver sinusoidal endothelial cells become enlarged and membrane permeability of hepatocytes becomes enhanced probably by the generation of membranous pores [45]. Intravenous injection of a volume corresponding to 8% of the body weight, which is probably equivalent to the total blood volume of a mouse [44], causes strong discomfort of the animals. Therefore, animal boards in some countries judge this treatment as too stressing for the animals, and deny the approval of such experiments.

Using hydrodynamic injection for the delivery of HBV genomes [15] allows the establishment of HBV replication at easily detectable levels. Viremia reached levels of 0.5–1 $\times$ 10^7 HBV/ml blood [15], comparable to titers observed following adenoviral genome transfer and to that in acutely infected humans. HBV transcripts were detected the day after the in vivo transfection, replicative intermediates shortly thereafter. Replication levels were stable between days 4 and 7 post-injection, decreased after day 7 and became undetectable at day 15 post-injection [15]. The efficacy of a gene transfer by hydrodynamic injection shows a relatively high variability [45] most likely resulting in variable levels of HBV replication. Despite the relatively short term of HBV replication observed, the immune response against HBV can be monitored.

In summary, in the last few years major advances in the development of models have been achieved which allow to study the onset and establishment of HBV infection and to characterize the immune response during acute infection in more detail. Either by hydrodynamic injection or with the help of adenoviral vectors, replication-competent HBV genomes are transferred into mouse hepatocytes where they establish an HBV replication at levels comparable to an acute hepatitis B in humans. In both systems, replication is controlled by the host immune response which becomes evident by the appearance of T cells and antibodies recognizing HBV antigens prior to the decrease and later on disappearance of HBV replication.

These systems will allow studying viral dynamics in a tightly controlled in vivo system. They allow comparing the fitness of natural and engineered viral mutants and to study the HBV replication cycle in vivo. In the constructs used, HBV replication is initiated exclusively under control of the endogenous HBV promoters. This allows investigations of the replication competence of viral mutants and the function of regulatory viral proteins on the viral life cycle by carefully directed knockouts. Furthermore, the use of genetically modified mice whose immunoregulatory or immune effector functions have been deleted or overexpressed allow to further dissect the immune response to the virus. However, unlike in natural infection, a constant proportion of the hepatocytes are 'infected' at the same time since mice do not support the spread of HBV. Whether this results in distinct differences concerning the immune response to HBV needs to be determined.

Acknowledgements

The authors thank Heinz Schaller for stimulating discussions and continuous support. The work was supported by the Deutsche Forschungsgemeinschaft, grant PR 618/2.

References

1 WHO: Viral Hepatitis Prevention Board: Prevention and Control of Hepatitis B in the Community. WHO Communicable Series No 1 1996;1–26.
2 Hoofnagle JH, di Bisceglie A: The treatment of chronic viral hepatitis. N Engl J Med 1997; 336:347–56.

3 Zuckerman AJ, Lavanchy D: Treatment options for chronic hepatitis. Antivirals look promising. BMJ 1999;319:799–800.
4 Summers J, Mason WS: Replication of the genome of a hepatitis B-like virus by reverse transcription of an RNA intermediate. Cell 1982;29:403–415.
5 Ganem D, Schneider R: Hepadnaviridae: The viruses and their replication; in Knipe DM, Howley PM (eds): Fields Virology, ed 4. Philadelphia, Lippincott Williams & Wilkins, 2001, vol 2, pp 2923–2970.
6 Nassal M, Schaller H: Hepatitis B virus replication – An update. J Viral Hepat 1996;3:217–226.
7 Loser P, Sandig V, Kirillova I, Strauss M: Evaluation of HBV promoters for use in hepatic gene therapy. Biol Chem Hoppe Seyler 1996;377:187–193.
8 Gripon P, Rumin S, Urban S, Le Seyec J, Glaise D, Cannie I, Guyomard C, Lucas J, Trepo C, Guguen-Guillouzo C: Infection of a human hepatoma cell line by hepatitis B virus. Proc Natl Acad Sci USA 2002;99:15655–15660.
9 Guidotti LG, Matzke B, Schaller H, Chisari FV: High-level hepatitis B virus replication in transgenic mice. J Virol 1995;69:6158–6169.
10 Guidotti LG, Chisari FV: Noncytolytic control of viral infections by the innate and adaptive immune response. Annu Rev Immunol 2001;19:65–91.
11 Eto T, Takahashi H: Enhanced inhibition of hepatitis B virus production by asialoglycoprotein receptor-directed interferon. Nat Med 1999;5:577–581.
12 Feitelson MA, DeTolla LJ, Zhou XD: A chronic carrier-like state is established in nude mice injected with cloned hepatitis B virus DNA. J Virol 1988;62:1408–1415.
13 Takahashi H, Fujimoto J, Hanada S, Isselbacher KJ: Acute hepatitis in rats expressing human hepatitis B virus transgenes. Proc Natl Acad Sci USA 1995;92:1470–1474.
14 Sprinzl MF, Oberwinkler H, Schaller H, Protzer U: Transfer of hepatitis B virus genome by adenovirus vectors into cultured cells and mice: Crossing the species barrier. J Virol 2001;75: 5108–5118.
15 Yang PL, Althage A, Chung J, Chisari FV: Hydrodynamic injection of viral DNA: A mouse model of acute hepatitis B virus infection. Proc Natl Acad Sci USA 2002;99:13825–13830.
16 Ren S, Nassal M: Hepatitis B virus (HBV) virion and covalently closed circular DNA formation in primary tupaia hepatocytes and human hepatoma cell lines upon HBV genome transduction with replication-defective adenovirus vectors. J Virol 2001;75:1104–1116.
17 Sprinzl MF, Dumortier J, Protzer U: Construction of recombinant adenoviruses that produce infectious HBV; in Hamatke R, Lau J (eds): Hepatitis B Virus Protocols. Methods in Molecular Medicine. Totowa, Humana Press, 2003, vol 1, pp 209–218.
18 Delaney IV WE, Isom HC: Hepatitis B virus replication in human HepG2 cells mediated by hepatitis B virus recombinant baculovirus. Hepatology 1998;28:1134–1146.
19 Ragot T, Opolon P, Perricaudet M: Adenoviral gene delivery. Methods Cell Biol 1997;52:229–260.
20 Bramson JL, Graham FL, Gauldie J: The use of adenoviral vectors for gene therapy and gene transfer in vivo. Curr Opin Biotechnol 1995;6:590–595.
21 Li Q, Kay MA, Finegold M, Stratford-Perricaudet LD, Woo SL: Assessment of recombinant adenoviral vectors for hepatic gene therapy. Hum Gene Ther 1993;4:403–409.
22 Hegenbarth S, Gerolami R, Protzer U, Tran PL, Brechot C, Gerken G, Knolle PA: Liver sinusoidal endothelial cells are not permissive for adenovirus type 5. Hum Gene Ther 2000;11:481–486.
23 Delaney WE IV, Miller TG, Isom HC: Use of the hepatitis B virus recombinant baculovirus-HepG2 system to study the effects of (–)-β-2′,3′-dideoxy-3′-thiacytidine on replication of hepatitis B virus and accumulation of covalently closed circular DNA. Antimicrob Agents Chemother 1999;43: 2017–2026.
24 Hofmann C, Sandig V, Jennings G, Rudolph M, Schlag P, Strauss M: Efficient gene transfer into human hepatocytes by baculovirus vectors. Proc Natl Acad Sci USA 1995;92:10099–10103.
25 Boyce FM, Bucher NLR: Baculovirus-mediated transfer into mammalian cells. Proc Natl Acad Sci USA 1996;93:2348–2352.
26 Hofmann C, Strauss M: Baculovirus-mediated gene transfer in the presence of human serum or blood facilitated by inhibition of the complement system. Gene Ther 1998;5:531–536.
27 Graham FL, Smiley J, Russel WC, Nairn R: Characteristics of a human cell line transformed by DNA from human adenovirus type 5. J Gen Virol 1977;36:59–72.

28 Petersen J, Dandri M, Gupta S, Rogler CE: Liver repopulation with xenogenic hepatocytes in B and T cell-deficient mice leads to chronic hepadnavirus infection and clonal growth of hepatocellular carcinoma. Proc Natl Acad Sci USA 1998;95:310–315.
29 Ohashi K, Marion PL, Nakai H, Meuse L, Cullen JM, Bordier BB, Schwall R, Greenberg HB, Glenn JS, Kay MA: Sustained survival of human hepatocytes in mice: A model for in vivo infection with human hepatitis B and hepatitis delta viruses. Nat Med 2000;6:327–331.
30 Christ M, Lusky M, Stoeckel F, Dreyer D, Dieterle A, Michou AI, Pavirani A, Mehtali M: Gene therapy with recombinant adenovirus vectors: Evaluation of the host immune response. Immunol Lett 1997;57:19–25.
31 Ilan Y, Saito H, Thummala NR, Chowdhury NR: Adenovirus-mediated gene therapy of liver diseases. Semin Liver Dis 1999;19:49–59.
32 Kochanek S, Clemens PR, Mitani K, Chen HH, Chan S, Caskey CT: A new adenoviral vector: Replacement of all viral coding sequences with 28 kb of DNA independently expressing both full-length dystrophin and β-galactosidase. Proc Natl Acad Sci USA 1996;93:5731–5736.
33 Schiedner G, Morral N, Parks RJ, Wu Y, Koopmans SC, Langston C, Graham FL, Beaudet AL, Kochanek S: Genomic DNA transfer with a high-capacity adenovirus vector results in improved in vivo gene expression and decreased toxicity. Nat Genet 1998;18:180–183.
34 O'Neal WK, Zhou H, Morral N, Langston C, Parks RJ, Graham FL, Kochanek S, Beaudet AL: Toxicity associated with repeated administration of first-generation adenovirus vectors does not occur with a helper-dependent vector. Mol Med 2000;6:179–195.
35 Schödel F, Weimer T, Fernholz D, Schneider R, Sprengel R, Wildner G, Will H: The biology of avian hepatitis B viruses; in McLachlan A (ed): Molecular Biology of the Hepatitis B Virus. Boca Raton, CRC Press, 1991, pp 53–80.
36 Roggendorf M, Tolle TK: The woodchuck: An animal model for hepatitis B virus infection in man. Intervirology 1995;38:100–112.
37 Di Q, Summers J, Burch JB, Mason WS: Major differences between WHV and HBV in the regulation of transcription. Virology 1997;229:25–35.
38 Yan RQ, Su JJ, Huang DR, Gan YC, Yang C, Huang GH: Human hepatitis B virus and hepatocellular carcinoma. I. Experimental infection of tree shrews with hepatitis B virus. J Cancer Res Clin Oncol 1996;122:283–288.
39 Walter E, Keist R, Niederost B, Pult I, Blum HE: Hepatitis B virus infection of tupaia hepatocytes in vitro and in vivo. Hepatology 1996;24:1–5.
40 Brown JJ, Parashar B, Moshage H, Tanaka KE, Engelhardt D, Rabbani E, Roy-Chowdhury N, Roy-Chowdhury J: A long-term hepatitis B viremia model generated by transplanting nontumorigenic immortalized human hepatocytes in Rag-2-deficient mice. Hepatology 2000;31:173–181.
41 Dandri M, Burda MR, Torok E, Pollok JM, Iwanska A, Sommer G, Rogiers X, Rogler CE, Gupta S, Will H, Greten H, Petersen J: Repopulation of mouse liver with human hepatocytes and in vivo infection with hepatitis B virus. Hepatology 2001;33:981–988.
42 Will H, Cattaneo R, Darai G, Deinhardt F, Schellekens H, Schaller H: Infectious hepatitis B virus from cloned DNA of known nucleotide sequence. Proc Natl Acad Sci USA 1985;82:891–895.
43 Sprengel R, Kuhn C, Manso C, Will H: Cloned duck hepatitis B virus DNA is infectious in Peking ducks. J Virol 1984;52:932–937.
44 Liu F, Song Y, Liu D: Hydrodynamics-based transfection in animals by systemic administration of plasmid DNA. Gene Ther 1999;6:1258–1266.
45 Zhang G, Gao X, Song YK, Vollmer R, Stolz DB, Gasiorowski JZ, Dean DA, Liu D: Hydroporation as the mechanism of hydrodynamic delivery. Gene Ther 2004;11:1–8.

Ulrike Protzer, MD
Molekulare Infektiologie, Institut für Medizinische Mikrobiologie
Immunologie und Hygiene, Goldenfelsstrasse 19–21, DE–50935 Köln (Germany)
Tel. +49 221 4787285, Fax +49 221 4787288, E-Mail ulrike.protzer@uni-koeln.de

von Weizsäcker F, Roggendorf M (eds): Models of Viral Hepatitis.
Monogr Virol. Basel, Karger, 2005, vol 25, pp 42–55

Recent Advances in the Duck Hepatitis B Virus Model

Allison R. Jilbert[a,b]

[a]Hepatitis Virus Research Laboratory, Infectious Diseases Laboratories, Institute of Medical and Veterinary Science, Adelaide and [b]School of Molecular and Biomedical Science, University of Adelaide, North Terrace, Adelaide, S.A., Australia

Why Study Duck Hepatitis B Virus Infection?

Human hepatitis B virus (HBV) infection is a major worldwide health problem. Recent statistics from the World Health Organization indicate that 374 million people (6.4% of the world's population) have persistent HBV infection. Persistent infection results in a 25–50% lifetime risk of cirrhosis and primary liver cancer, leading to ~250,000–1,000,000 deaths per year from HBV-related liver disease [1]. The long-term objectives of our research are to design therapeutic strategies and to improve vaccines for human HBV infection. Our research is performed through study of Pekin ducks infected with duck hepatitis B virus (DHBV), a member of the *Avihepadnavirus* genus of the hepadnavirus family. DHBV-infected ducks and woodchuck hepatitis virus (WHV)-infected woodchucks have been studied as animal models for the human infection and have enhanced our understanding of the replication strategy, natural history, and pathogenesis of HBV infection.

The Avian Hepadnaviruses

The *Avihepadnavirus* genus includes DHBV isolated from Pekin ducks (*Anas domesticus*) [2], heron hepatitis B virus (HHBV) from grey herons (*Ardea cinerae*) [3], Ross goose hepatitis virus (RGHV) from Ross geese (*Anser rossii*) (Genebank DHBV-RGM 95589), snow goose hepatitis B virus

(SGHBV) from snow geese (*Anser caerulescens*) [4], stork hepatitis B virus (STHBV) from white storks (*Ciconia ciconia*) [5], the Australian maned duck, (MDHBV), and grey teal (GTHBV) hepatitis B viruses [R.J. Dixon, pers. commun.].

The avihepadnaviruses have been classified phylogenetically into 'Chinese' and 'Western' isolates as well as four highly distinct lineages that include the SGHBV, RGHV, STHBV and HHBV [4, 6, 7]. Nucleotide sequence divergence within the 'Chinese' and 'Western' DHBV strains is 5.99 and 3.35% while divergence between the strains is 9.8% [7].

Species Specificity of Hepadnavirus Infection

All of the hepadnaviruses share similar features of genome and virion structure and replicate by reverse transcription in the cytoplasm of infected cells using an RNA intermediate. However, despite being members of the same virus family, they are generally not able to cross-infect. Their species specificity is determined by binding of the viral surface protein (part of the viral envelope) to specific receptors located on the surface of host cells. Receptor binding is followed by receptor-mediated virus uptake and infection. Thus only hosts with similar receptors can be infected with the same or closely related viruses.

The cell specificity of DHBV infection is determined by the presence of specific receptors for virus binding and entry into hepatocytes, the major cell type infected. In early studies, cell surface receptors on primary duck hepatocytes were shown to bind DHBV particles in a species-specific manner [8]. Receptor binding occurs via peptides encoded by the DHBV envelope protein, also called surface antigen (DHBsAg) and is followed by cell entry via endocytosis. Recent studies have determined that carboxypeptidase D (180 kDa) is capable of binding DHBsAg particles with high affinity [9]. The organ distribution of the DHBV-binding activity mirrors the known sites of extrahepatic replication of DHBV and carboxypeptidase D is found on both internal and surface membranes of the cell. However, transfection of cells with carboxypeptidase D cDNA does not confer infectivity to DHBV [10], suggesting that other co-receptors or mechanisms may be operating. An additional DHBV-binding protein, glycine decarboxylase (120 kDa), has been identified [11, 12] and its cellular expression is restricted to the liver, kidney and pancreas, which are the three major organs of DHBV replication. These proteins are potential components of the DHBV receptor complex and probably have a role in determining DHBV organ tropism but the cellular receptor for DHBV is still unknown.

Features of DHBV Particles and Viral Replication

All members of the hepadnavirus family share similar features of genome and virion structure and possess an envelope, a nucleocapsid, a small, relaxed circular (RC) DNA genome and a carry a viral polymerase. The DHBV genome was originally thought to contain 3 open reading frames (ORF) and to lack an ORF encoding DHBV X protein. However, it was subsequently reported that avihepadnaviridae strains including HHBV [13] and later, DHBV [14] also have an X-ORF with X protein produced from an unconventional start codon. In addition to the X-ORF, hepadnaviruses also have an S-ORF, C-ORF, P-ORF encoding envelope, core and polymerase proteins.

The DHBV envelope is composed of a lipid bilayer containing 2 transmembrane forms of DHBsAg, the DHBV PreS/S and S proteins (36 and 17 kDa respectively). The DHBV nucleocapsid is icosahedral and composed of 180 or 240 copies of DHBV core protein (30 kDa). Both the surface and core proteins are highly immunogenic.

The DHBV genome ranges in size from 3,021 to 3,027 nt. The negative strand of the DHBV genome is nicked and has the viral polymerase molecule covalently attached to the 5′ end. Following infection of cells, and transport of the viral nucleocapsid to the nucleus, the RC DNA genome is converted to covalently closed circular DNA (cccDNA). Host cell enzymes then use the cccDNA template to produce viral pre-genomic and messenger RNAs. RNA synthesis is followed by transport of RNA to the cytoplasm, production of core and polymerase proteins and assembly of viral nucleocapsids containing pre-genomic RNA. Viral DNA replication then occurs within the nucleocapsid using the viral polymerase (it functions as a reverse transcriptase) to copy pre-genomic RNA into single- and then partially double-stranded rcDNA genomes. Nucleocapsids containing mature RC DNA are enveloped by budding and leave the cell via the Golgi or are transported to the nucleus to form a pool of super-coiled cccDNA [15, 16]. DHBV infected cells contain 6–30 copies/cell of nuclear cccDNA and 160–500 copies of cytoplasmic single- and double-stranded replicative forms of DNA [17]. We recently showed that ΔHBV cccDNA is resistant to antiviral therapy and declines at a rate similar to the estimated rate of hepatocyte turnover [18].

DHBV-infected cells also contain integrated DHBV DNA sequences at a rate of ~1 copy in 10^3–10^4 cells [19]. This low rate of integration highlights that fact that, unlike retrovirus replication, where transcription of genomic RNA occurs from an integrated template, integration is a non-essential and infrequent event in hepadnavirus replication. Integrated DHBV DNA is usually monomeric and unable to act as template for production of the greater than genomic length pre-genomic RNA [19].

Experimental Models for Studying HBV Infection

Treatment of persistent HBV infection has proved difficult because of the stability of viral cccDNA, which forms a viral 'reservoir' within infected cells, and the lack of animal models with well-characterized immune systems that can be used to develop new therapeutic strategies. To address this problem, HBV transgenic mice were developed and have been used to demonstrate cytokine-mediated suppression of HBV replication following injection of HBV-specific T lymphocytes. However, because hepadnavirus infection is highly species-specific, mice are not naturally susceptible to HBV and therefore do not provide a system for studying initiation or resolution of infection. Also, HBV transgenic mice do not produce cccDNA, so effects of cytokines on cccDNA and the fate of cells containing cccDNA cannot be studied in this model. Studies of the resolution of HBV infection must therefore be performed in humans by collecting blood and liver samples, or in animals susceptible to human HBV (e.g. chimpanzees) or that can be infected with other, similar members of the hepadnavirus family (e.g. ducks and woodchucks).

DHBV-Infected Ducks as a Model for Human HBV Infection

Hepadnaviruses have the ability to cause either transient or persistent infections. The outcome of infection is strongly age-dependent and is also related to the viral dose. In humans, persistent HBV infection develops in most individuals infected with HBV at or around the time of birth, but only in 5–10% of HBV-infected adults. Similar age-related outcomes are seen in DHBV infection: Persistent DHBV infection occurs following either congenital transmission of virus (from the bloodstream of the female duck to the yolk sac and liver of the developing embryo) [17] or following experimental transmission of DHBV (by intravenous or intramuscular inoculation) to newly hatched ducklings [20]. In contrast, infection of older ducks usually results in transient DHBV infection [21].

In ducks with persistent DHBV infection, viral replication occurs mainly in the liver with high levels of DHBV replication and antigen expression in the cytoplasm of most, if not all hepatocytes. High numbers of DHBV and 'empty' surface antigen containing particles are released into the bloodstream. Titers in the bloodstream may reach 1×10^{10} DHBV particles and 1×10^{13} surface antigen particles per millilter of serum [20]. Due to the large numbers of DHBV particles circulating in the bloodstream of infected ducks, DHBV infection is readily transmitted by intravenous or parenteral inoculation of infected blood.

Specific Infectivity Rates of HBV and DHBV Infection

HBV infection is readily transmitted by needle stick injury and sexual transmission suggesting that only a small number of viral particles are required for transmission. Since HBV and DHBV have many similar structural features, and because the infectivity of HBV could not be determined using cell culture systems, we performed titration experiments with the Australian strain of DHBV in newly hatched ducks and found they could be infected and developed persistent infection after inoculation with just one viral particle [20]. This finding has been used as a reference point for viral receptor-binding studies, since it provides assurance that most of the virions present in infectious stocks are intact and infectious.

Experimental inoculation of newly hatched ducks has also provided a system for study of the kinetics of virus growth in the liver where wild-type DHBV infection has been shown to spread rapidly from cell-to-cell with a doubling time of 16 h resulting in full infection of the liver from a single virus particle within 4 weeks [20]. Interestingly this timing is not unlike the incubation period of human HBV infection where HBV DNA and HBV surface antigen are detected in the bloodstream within 4–6 weeks after infection.

Use of the DHBV Model to Study Virulence Determinants

The DHBV model has also been used to study the kinetics of growth of specific viral mutants in vivo including DHBV strains with mutations in the X-ORF [14] and cytopathic mutants of DHBV with specific mutations in the viral preS protein [22–24]. The overall aim of the work was to investigate how different hepadnavirus proteins affect the course of infection and the type of disease produced. Studies were performed with a German DHBV strain with a mutation in the ORF of the X protein, a viral transactivator; and the DHBV16 wild-type strain, with a mutation in the PreS/S protein that forms part of the viral envelope. Studies involved comparison of the in vivo growth of the mutants with their wild-type strain using, as reference, previously determined growth rates, infectivity and infection outcomes of with the Australian strain of DHBV [20].

Studies of a DHBV X Protein Knockout Strain

Hepadnavirus X proteins have reported effects on signal transduction, transcription, transformation, cell proliferation and the development of liver cancer. In recent in vivo experiments using WHV strains with X-ORF mutations, transient infection with reversion to wild type was seen, suggesting an important role for X protein in vivo [25]. In recent studies in our laboratory, newly hatched ducks were used to test whether the DHBx protein plays a role in virus infection by comparing the in vivo infectivity and growth characteristics of a DHBV3 strain with a stop codon in the X-like ORF (DHBV3-X-KO) to those of the wild-type strain. We compared the in vivo infectivity and growth characteristics of this mutant to wild-type DHBV3. Stocks of DHBV3 or DHBV3-X-KO virus had comparable infectious titers (ID_{50}), with 1 infectious particle to 18 DNA genomes for DHBV3, and 4 DNA genomes for DHBV3-X-KO [24]. The ability of both strains to induce infection that resulted in stable viremia, and the kinetics of virus spread in the liver following inoculation of ducklings with 1,500 ID_{50}, was also similar. Under controlled age/dose conditions, a similar percentage of ducks inoculated with DHBV3 and DHBV3-X-KO developed persistent infection. Thus, none of the infection parameters assayed were detectably affected by the X ORF knockout mutation allowing us to demonstrate that the DHBV X-ORF is not required for viral infection and replication in vivo [24]. This finding allowed us to resolve the current controversy about the role of the hepadnavirus X protein in vivo.

Studies of a Cytopathic Mutant of DHBV

The DHBV PreS/S envelope protein is required for assembly of enveloped virus particles and has been shown to regulate the intracellular amplification of covalently closed circular DNA (cccDNA). In collaboration with Jesse Summers (University of New Mexico) we compared the growth of the DHBV16 wild-type strain to a cytopathic DHBV mutant (G133E), with a single amino acid codon change at residue 133 in the PreS/S protein. Stocks of DHBV16 or G133E had similar amounts of DHBV DNA and DHBsAg and had similar ratios of DNA genomes/infectious particle that were 25- (G133E) and 50-fold (DHBV16) lower than AusDHBV [20]. Short-term one-step infection experiments conducted in 1-day-old ducks inoculated with 5×10^8 ID_{50} demonstrated that infection with G133E led to increased levels of cccDNA, and aspartate transaminase levels four times the upper limit of normal by 95 h post-inoculation (pi). Ducklings inoculated with 1,500 ID_{50} of DHBV16 or G133E were used to study the cell-to-cell spread of virus within the liver. Delays were observed in the rate of spread of G133E infection compared to wild type at each time point, reaching full infection of >95% of hepatocytes in the wild-type and G133E-infected ducks by day 6 and 7 pi respectively. Both viruses showed a characteristic pattern of spread from single isolated infected cells to groups of cells. The content of total intrahepatic viral DNA was similar with both wild type and mutant, while the level of cccDNA was consistently 4- to 6-fold higher with G133E. Apoptotic cells were seen more frequently with the mutant infection than wild type from days 7–13 pi and bile duct proliferation and acinar regeneration of hepatocytes were more extensive with G133E from days 5–12 pi. These studies confirmed that point mutation in the viral envelope protein led to increased accumulation of cccDNA, slower spread of virus to adjacent cells, and evidence for increased apoptosis, cell death and cell regeneration, in comparison to wild-type virus [24; Meier et al., unpubl. data].

The Role of the Immune Response in DHBV Infection

Human HBV infection shows age-related outcomes with 90–95% of neonates developing persistent infection, whilst in adults the rate of persistent infection is around 5–10%. It has been proposed that the failure of >90% of neonates to recover from HBV infection is linked to maturity of the immune system and inability of the host to mount effective immune responses. We thus studied the different age-related outcomes of DHBV infection and found similar outcomes to HBV. As with HBV infection, increasing the age of ducks at the time of DHBV inoculation led to resolution rather than the development of persistent infection [17, 21]. In older ducks the outcome of infection is linked to the dose of virus inoculated. For example, inoculation of 1×10^6 genomes of DHBV into 14-day-old ducks leads to a persistent infection while inoculation of 4×10^4 genomes results in transient infection [21]. Even very high doses (up to 2×10^{11} viral particles) normally cause only transient infection in adult ducks [21]. The failure to develop persistent infection in older ducks is not due to a loss of receptors or to an inability to infect hepatocytes in the liver of older ducks since the ducks receiving 2×10^{11} genomes had DHBV infection in >95% of hepatocytes at days 6, 9 and 12 after inoculation [21]. It is thought that older ducks more effectively generate immune responses resulting in production of virus neutralizing antibodies and cytotoxic T lymphocytes that enable resolution of DHBV infection [26].

Definition of the different outcomes of DHBV infection in ducks of different ages inoculated with defined doses of virus allow us to use the DHBV model to design experiments with predictable outcomes and to test antiviral and immunotherapies designed to alter the outcome of infection. This work forms the basis ongoing vaccine and antiviral studies in the laboratory outlined below.

Liver Damage and Persistent DHBV Infection

The DHBV model is being used to study the role of the immune response in determining the outcome of DHBV infection. Since hepadnavirus infection is non-cytopathic, the liver damage seen during DHBV infection results from the immune response directed against infected cells. Persistent infection with avian hepadnaviruses generally results in a mild hepatitis that does not usually progress to liver disease or to cirrhosis or hepatocellular carcinoma (HCC) [27, 28]. The liver disease seen in persistent DHBV infection is similar to the 'healthy' carrier status of humans infected with HBV, which can last for several decades. The failure to detect liver disease, cirrhosis and HCC in persistently DHBV-infected ducks may to be linked to the timing and mode of transmission of these viruses since they are usually transmitted vertically by in ovo transmission resulting in congenital infection with immune tolerance and an absence of, or only mild, liver disease [17, 27, 28]. In support of this idea, experimental infection of 4-month-old ducks with DHBV leads to the development of persistent DHBV infections with mild and marked liver disease [21] and these animals may have a greater chance of developing HCC. The ability of DHBV-infected ducks to progress to HCC may also be affected by their limited life span. Pekin ducks with persistent DHBV infection have been studied for many years without the appearance of HCC [29, 30]. HCC has been however detected in ducks in a Chinese province where aflatoxin exposure was common [31].

The Role of the Immune Response in the Resolution of Transient DHBV Infection

A major focus of our current research is to determine the factors that allow the host to resolve viral infection and to develop immunity to re-infection. To do this we have developed ELISA assays to detect antibody responses during DHBV infection and we are characterizing cellular immune responses using antigen-specific in vitro proliferation assays and analysis of cytokine gene expression by RT-PCR. Understanding of the age-related effects and the role of the immune response in the resolution of infection would provide a framework for addressing the clinically important issue of why some patients, but not others, remain persistently infected. This is also of fundamental importance for designing and testing approaches for immunotherapy of patients with persistent HBV infection.

Although in our previous studies we have shown that resolution of DHBV infection in 4-month-old ducks is accompanied by moderate inflammatory changes in the liver [22], there are as yet no studies of the extent of spread of infection in immune competent ducks, the timing of resolution, and the contributions of cell death vs. possible cytokine-mediated curing of infected cells. Our current work aims to define the timing of transient DHBV infection, the extent of cell-to-cell spread, and the variability between infected animals, particularly because the ducks we use are not inbred. Based on these results, we will then proceed to a detailed determination of the amount of hepatocyte death and regeneration that accompanies resolution of transient DHBV infection. The studies include experimental inoculation of ducks with DHBV followed by determination of the timing of cell-mediated immune responses, appearance of viremia, anti-surface antibodies and immune complexes, the number, location and state of activation of Kupffer cells, the resident macrophages of the liver and the cellular location within in each liver lobule of HBV-infected and apoptotic hepatocytes, infiltrating lymphocytes and Kupffer cells.

We hypothesize that both humoral and cell-mediated immune responses, coupled with the ability of liver cells to divide to replace cells that have died, enables the resolution of hepadnavirus infections without a life-threatening crisis of liver destruction. We also hypothesize that immune-mediated cell death plays a major role in the resolution of transient HBV infections by promoting regeneration of liver cells leading to loss of replicative intermediates and to loss or dilution of cccDNA and that antiviral antibodies are critical for resolution as they lead to virus neutralization and protect newly divided cells from re-infection.

In the past, our ability to study the role of cell-mediated immune responses and cytokine-mediated curing of infected cells has been limited by a lack of reagents for assaying cellular markers and cytokine expression in ducks. This has now changed. We have developed a series of assays for monitoring viral antigen-specific T-cell proliferation in vitro [32] and cDNA clones for duck interferon (IFN)-α [33], IFN-γ [34, 35] are now available. In addition a new series of cDNA clones for duck T-lymphocyte and cellular markers (including CD3 ε, CD4, CD8, MHC I and II: *Anas platyrhynchos* T-cell receptor CD3 ε chain mRNA, GenBank AF378704; T-cell surface glycoprotein CD4 precursor mRNA, GenBank AF378701; T-cell antigen CD8 α mRNA, GenBank AF378373; MHC class I antigen α chain mRNA, GenBank AF393511; MHC class II antigen β chain mRNA, GenBank AF390589) have been provided by Prof. David Higgins (University of Hong Kong), and we have recently developed RT-PCR assays for detection of duck IFN-α, IFN-γ, CD3, CD4, and CD8 and using duck B-actin and GAPDH [Reaiche et al., unpubl. data] as controls. We have also developed an ELISPOT assay for duck IFN-γ using anti-chicken IFN-γ monoclonal antibodies, 9.1 [35]. Monoclonal antibodies to duck CD4 and CD8 are also available from Ursula Schultz (University of Freiburg) and monoclonal antibodies to duck thrombocytes have been produced by Edward Bertram [36]. Use of the duck model, with increased numbers of animals, will allow us to study the rate of turnover of infected cells during resolution transient infection by incorporating bromodeoxyuridine into dividing cells. This will give us a measure of the rate of division of cells that in the WHV and HBV models can only be determined indirectly using Tunel or PCNA assays.

Our interest in the duck model is based in part on our recent studies of the role of cell death and regeneration and immune responses in the resolution of transient WHV infections. In studies of WHV, resolution of infection was accompanied by cell death and turnover of hepatocytes resulting in at least one entire liver of hepatocytes being destroyed and regenerated during resolution [37]. Analysis of integrated WHV DNA indicated that the recovered liver was populated by previously infected hepatocytes that had undergone cell division, consistent with the idea that loss of virus infection from individual hepatocytes required turnover of infected cells [37]. Resolution of infection was also accompanied by activation of Kupffer cells, marked apoptosis and inflammation. The Kupffer cell population in the liver increased from 5–9% (at weeks 0–4 after infection) to 25–29% of total lobular cells (at weeks 8–12). Kupffer cells also accumulated PAS-diastase-resistant material and dramatically increased in size. The high fraction of PAS-D-positive Kupffer cells and high levels of apoptosis suggested that a major proportion of the hepatocyte population had been destroyed by the host immune response [Jilbert et al., unpubl. data]. Studies of ducks during the resolution of transient DHBV infections also show Kupffer cell activation, suggesting that cell death is also occurring in this model [Jilbert et al., unpubl. data].

Virus Infection Persists after the Apparent Resolution of Transient DHBV Infection

Originally, it was thought that recovery from transient hepadnavirus infection involved complete elimination of the virus. However, recent work by our laboratory and others has revealed that this is not the case. Studies with DHBV and WHV models and observations in human patients indicate that low-level infection persists after recovery and can be reactivated in certain circumstances. The presence of this low-level residual virus infection may be linked to the HCC that sometimes occurs in humans and woodchucks that have recovered from transient infection. Nonetheless, because HCC occurs at a much lower incidence than in individuals with high-level persistent infection, achieving such a level of control of infection would be a major breakthrough in HBV research. Little is known about the molecular state, levels of expression, and cellular location of residual hepadnavirus infections. Our studies of residual DHBV infection [38, 39; Le Mire et al., unpubl. data] suggest that viral DNA replication is highly repressed and that most viral DNA is present in the form of cccDNA. Experiments are therefore proposed to determine how and where residual infections are maintained, how they are controlled, and why they fail to rapidly rebound. Inducing a permanent suppression of virus, as occurs naturally during recovery from transient infections, would reduce the ultimate risk of serious liver disease.

Combining Antiviral and Novel DNA Vaccines for Treatment of Persistent HBV Infections

We have tested the immunogenicity and protective effects of DNA vaccines expressing DHBV surface antigens in adult and newly hatched ducks and have found that DNA vaccination induces high levels of anti-surface antibodies accompanied by full or partial protection against DHBV challenge [40; Miller et al., unpubl. data]. We have also conducted studies and have proved the hypothesis that a transient or persistent outcome of hepadnavirus infection is determined by the balance between the rates of virus replication and induction of immune responses during a critical period in acute infection. These studies were conducted using antiviral treatment with the Bristol-Myers Squibb compound, entecavir (ETV), previously shown to be highly effective against DHBV infection in vivo [41]. In our studies, treatment of ducks with ETV during the early stages of acute infection did not prevent DHBV infection of the liver, but reduced levels of virus replication and the spread of infection resulting in transient rather than persistent DHBV infection [Foster et al., unpubl. data]. This finding provides the experimental basis for the use of post-exposure antiviral therapy in altering the outcome of HBV infection in humans.

We also tested the ability of DNA vaccines expressing DHBV surface antigens to protect newly hatched ducks from the development of persistent infection. DNA vaccination prior to virus challenge did not result in detectable levels of anti-surface antibodies prior to challenge, but led to reduced numbers of infected hepatocytes early after challenge and resulted in transient rather than persistent infection in 5 out of 6 vaccinated ducklings inoculated with 5×10^7 genomes while all 6 control ducklings developed persistent DHBV infection [Miller et al., unpubl. data]. These studies indicated that the ability of the immune system to resolve DHBV infection is linked to the dose of virus inoculated, the number of hepatocytes initially infected and the rate of spread of infection within the liver. The results also suggested that DNA vaccines provide a realistic alternative to conventional subunit vaccines for inducing protective immune responses in young animals [Miller et al., unpubl. data].

New treatment strategies for persistent DHBV infection are being developed using ETV, to reduce viral load, and vaccination with DNA vaccines expressing DHBV antigens. In our first combination antiviral and DNA vaccine study [18], ETV treatment reduced levels of viral replication and antigen expression in the liver and serum. However, the administration of 5 doses of DNA vaccine expressing the DHBV S, PreS/S and core antigens did not prevent rebound of DHBV infection or have long-term beneficial effects. We are attempting to enhance the immune response by using whole-cell DNA vaccines composed of primary duck embryonic fibroblasts transfected with plasmid

DNA expressing DHBcAg, an internal antigen of the virus. We are also developing DNA vaccine prime, and recombinant fowl poxvirus boost protocols for treatment of persistent DHBV infection.

Acknowledgements

The research described herein was conducted in the hepatitis virus research laboratory at the Institute of Medical and Veterinary Science and the University of Adelaide and was funded by the National Health and Medical Research Council of Australia, Institute of Medical and Veterinary Science and the University of Adelaide. The author is indebted to present and past colleagues from the laboratory with particular mention of Darren Miller, Catherine Scougall, Edward Bertram, Wendy Foster, Marc Le Mire, Philip Meier, Georget Reaiche, Chris Burrell and Ieva Kotlarski. Studies of WHV infection have been performed in collaboration with William Mason (Fox Chase Cancer Centre) and Jesse Summers (University of New Mexico).

References

1 Huang MA, Lok AS: Natural history of hepatitis B and outcomes after liver transplantation. Clin Liver Dis 2003;7:521–536.

2 Mason WS, Seal G, Summers J: Virus of Pekin ducks with structural and biological relatedness to human hepatitis B virus. J Virol 1980;36:829–836.

3 Sprengel R, Kaleta EF, Will H: Isolation and characterization of a hepatitis B virus endemic in herons. J Virol 1988;62:3832–3839.

4 Chang SF, Netter HJ, Bruns M, Schneider R, Frölich K, Will H: A new avian hepadnavirus infecting snow geese (*Anser caerulescens*) produces a significant fraction of virions containing single-stranded DNA. Virology 1999;262:39–54.

5 Pult I, Netter HJ, Bruns M, Prassolov A, Sirma H, Hohenberg H, Chang SF, Frolich K, Krone O, Kaleta EF, Will H: Identification and analysis of a new hepadnavirus in white storks. Virology 2001;289:114–128.

6 Triyatni M, Ey PL, Tran H, Le Mire M, Qiao M, Burrell CJ, Jilbert AR: Sequence comparison of an Australian duck hepatitis B virus strain with other avian hepadnaviruses. J Gen Virol 2001;82:373–378.

7 Mangisa NP, Smuts HE, Kramvis A, Linley CW, Skelton M, Tucker TJ, de la M Hall P, Kahn D, Jilbert AR, Kew MC: Molecular characterization of duck hepatitis B virus isolates from South African ducks. Virus Genes 2004;28:181–188.

8 Pugh JC, Di Q, Mason WS, Simmons H: Susceptibility to duck hepatitis B virus infection is associated with the presence of cell surface receptor sites that efficiently bind viral particles. J Virol 1995;69:4814–4822.

9 Kuroki K, Cheung R, Marion PL, Ganem D: A cell surface protein that binds avian hepatitis B virus particles. J Virol 1994;68:2091–2096.

10 Breiner KM, Urban S, Schaller H: Carboxypeptidase D (gp180), a Golgi-resident protein, functions in the attachment and entry of avian hepatitis B viruses. J Virol 1998;72: 8098–8104.

11 Li JS, Tong SP, Wands JR: Characterization of a 120-kDa Pre-S-binding protein as a candidate duck hepatitis B virus receptor. J Virol 1996;70:6029–6035.

12 Li J, Tong S, Wands JR: Identification and expression of glycine decarboxylase (p120) as a duck hepatitis B virus pre-S envelope-binding protein. J Biol Chem 1999;274:27658–27665.

13 Netter HJ, Chassot S, Chang SF, Cova, L, Will H: Sequence heterogeneity of heron hepatitis B virus genomes determined by full-length DNA amplification and direct sequencing reveals novel and unique features. J Gen Virol 1997;78:1707–1718.
14 Chang SF, Netter HJ, Hildt E, Schuster R, Schaefer S, Hsu YC, Rang A, Will H: Duck hepatitis B virus expresses a regulatory HBx-like protein from a hidden open reading frame. J Virol 2001; 75:161–170.
15 Bock CT, Schwinn S, Locarnini S, Fyfe J, Manns M, Trautwein C, Zentgraf H: Structural organisation of the HBV minichromosome. J Mol Biol 2001;307:183–196.
16 Newbold JE, Xin H, Tencza M, Sherman G, Dean J, Bowden S, Locarnini S: The covalently closed duplex form of the hepadnavirus genome exists in situ as a heterogeneous population of viral minichromosomes. J Virol 1995;69:3350–3357.
17 Jilbert AR, Wu T, England J, Hall PM, Carp N, O'Connell A, Mason WS: Rapid resolution of DHBV infections occurs after massive hepatocellular involvement. J Virol 1992;66:1377–1388.
18 Foster WK, Miller DS, Marion PL, Colonno RJ, Kotlarski I, Jilbert AR: Entecavir therapy combined with DNA vaccination for persistent duck hepatitis B virus infection. Antimicrobial Agents Chemother 2003;47:2624–2635.
19 Yang W, Summers J: Integration of hepadnavirus DNA in infected liver: Evidence for a linear precursor. J Virol 1999;73:9710–9717.
20 Jilbert AR, Miller DS, Scougall CA, Turnbull HT, Burrell CJ: Kinetics of duck hepatitis B virus infection following low dose virus inoculation: One virus DNA genome is infectious in neonatal ducks. Virology 1996;226:338–345.
21 Jilbert AR, Botten JD, Miller DS, Bertram E, Hall P de la M, Kotlarski I, Burrell CJ: Characterisation of age- and dose-related outcomes of duck hepatitis B virus infection. Virology 1998;244:273–282.
22 Lenhoff RJ, Luscombe CA, Summers J: Competition in vivo between a cytopathic variant and a wild-type duck hepatitis B virus. Virology 1998;251:85–95.
23 Lenhoff RJ, Luscombe CA, Summers J: Acute liver injury following infection with a cytopathic strain of duck hepatitis B virus. Hepatology 1999;29:563–571.
24 Meier P, Scougall CA, Burrell CJ, Jilbert AR: Analysis of infectivity and in vivo growth characteristics of a cytopathic duck hepatitis mutant, G133E. Proc 11th International Symposium of Viral Hepatitis and Liver Disease, 2004; in press.
25 Zhang Z, Torii N, Hu Z, Jacob J, Liang TJ: X-deficient woodchuck hepatitis virus mutants behave like attenuated viruses and induce protective immunity in vivo. J Clin Invest 2001;108: 1523–1531.
26 Jilbert AR, Kotlarski I: Immune responses to duck hepatitis B virus infection. Dev Comp Immunol 2000;24:285–302.
27 Marion PL, Knight SS, Hot BK, Guo YY, Robinson WS, Popper H: Liver disease associated with duck hepatitis B virus infection of domestic ducks. Proc Natl Acad Sci USA 1984;81:898–902.
28 Marion PL, Cullen JM, Azcarraga RR, Van Davelaar MJ, Robinson WS: Experimental transmission of duck hepatitis B virus to Pekin ducks and domestic geese. Hepatology 1987;7:724–731.
29 Cova L, Wild CP, Mehrotra R, Turusov V, Shirai T, Lambert V, Jacquet C, Tomatis L, Trepo C, Montesano R: Contribution of aflatoxin B1 and hepatitis B virus infection in the induction of liver tumors in ducks. Cancer Res 1990;50:2156–2163.
30 Cullen JM, Marion PL, Sherman GJ, Hong X, Newbold JE: Hepatic neoplasms in aflatoxin B1-treated, congenital duck hepatitis B virus-infected and virus-free Pekin ducks. Cancer Res 1990;50:4072–4080.
31 Cova L, Mehrotra R, Wild CP, Chutimataewin S, Cao SF, Duflot A, Prave M, Yu SZ, Montesano R, Trepo C: Duck hepatitis B virus infection, aflatoxin B1 and liver cancer in domestic Chinese ducks. Br J Cancer 1994;69:104–109.
32 Miller DS, Bertram EM, Scougall CA, Kotlarski I, Jilbert AR: Studying host immune responses against duck hepatitis B virus infection; in Hamanake RK, Lau JYN (ed): Methods in Molecular Medicine. Hepatitis B and D Protocols. Totowa, Humana Press, 2004, vol 96, pp 3–28.
33 Schultz U, Kock J, Schlicht HJ, Staeheli P: Recombinant duck interferon: A new reagent for studying the mode of interferon action against HBV. Virology 1995;212:641–649.
34 Schultz U, Chisari FV: Recombinant duck interferon-γ inhibits DHBV replication in primary hepatocytes. J Virol 1999;73:3162–3168.

35 Huang A, Scougall CA, Lowenthal JW, Jilbert AR, Kotlarski I: Structural and functional homology between duck and chicken interferon-γ. Dev Comp Immunol 2001;25:55–68.
36 Bertram EM, Jilbert AR, Kotlarski I: Characterisation of thrombocytes purified from peripheral blood mononuclear cells of the duck. Res Vet Sci 1998;64:267–270.
37 Summers J, Jilbert AR, Yang W, Aldrich C, Saputelli J, Litwin S, Toll E, Mason WS: Hepatocyte turnover during resolution of a transient hepadnaviral infection. Proc Natl Acad Sci USA 2003;100:11652–11659.
38 Le Mire MF, Miller DS, Burrell CJ, Jilbert AR: Persistence of duck hepatitis B virus DNA after transient infection. J Gastroenterol Hepatol 2001;16(suppl):A78.
39 Le Mire MF, Miller DS, Foster W, Burrell CJ, Litwin S, Jilbert AR: Analysis of residual duck hepatitis B virus DNA after transient infection. Hepatology 2002;36:826A.
40 Triyatni M, Jilbert AR, Qiao M, Miller DS, Burrell CJ: Protective efficacy of yeast derived duck hepatitis B virus (DHBV) surface antigen proteins and DNA-based vaccines against DHBV infection. J Virol 1998;72:84–94.
41 Marion PL, Salazar FH, Winters MA, Colonno RJ: Potent efficacy of entecavir (BMS-200475) in a duck model of hepatitis B virus replication. Antimicrob Agents Chemother 2002;46:82–88.

Allison R. Jilbert
Hepatitis Virus Research Laboratory
Infectious Diseases Laboratories, Institute of Medical and Veterinary Science
PO Box 14 Rundle Mall, Adelaide, SA 5000 (Australia)
Tel. +61 8 8303 5399, Fax +61 8 8303 7532, E-Mail allison.jilbert@adelaide.edu.au

von Weizsäcker F, Roggendorf M (eds): Models of Viral Hepatitis.
Monogr Virol. Basel, Karger, 2005, vol 25, pp 56–65

Determinants of Hepadnaviral Species and Liver Cell Tropism

Anneke Funk, Li Lin, Mouna Mhamdi, Hans Will, Hüseyin Sirma

Department of General Virology, Heinrich-Pette-Institute for Experimental Virology and Immunology, University of Hamburg, Hamburg, Germany

Infections with the hepatitis B virus (HBV) remain a major medical challenge: 5% of the world's population are chronic carriers of the virus and have a high risk of developing liver diseases including cirrhosis or hepatocellular carcinoma. Despite the development of an effective and safe vaccine more than 20 years ago, the number of HBV infections has not declined and treatment with interferon-α and nucleoside analogs is still too inefficient or complicated by the emergence of drug-resistant mutants. To date, only very limited therapeutic options are available for treatment of HBV-associated liver cirrhosis and hepatocellular carcinoma.

Human HBV is the prototype of a small family of non-cytopathogenic, enveloped DNA viruses referred to as *Hepadnaviridae*. Other members of this family have been found in mammals such as woodchucks (WHV), ground squirrels (GSHV), and Arctic ground squirrels (AGSV) as well as in several bird species including ducks (DHBV) and grey herons (HHBV) [for a review, see 1]. Common features of hepadnaviruses include a similar genome organization and replication strategy as well as a rather strict host and liver tropism.

In the last two decades, the late steps of the hepadnaviral life cycle could be undeceived in considerable detail. In contrast, very little information is available on the infectious entry pathway. The cellular partners involved in cell-virus interactions at this early stage of infection have remained unidentified and the molecular determinants of host specificity, hepatotropism and the nature of the receptor complex still await their discovery. Studies addressing the early steps of the hepadnaviral life cycle were mainly hampered by the lack of reliable cell lines and small animal models permissive for HBV. A complete viral infection cycle mimicking natural HBV infection in vitro can be achieved only in primary human hepatocytes. The disadvantages of this system are restricted accessibility to the cells as well as inefficiency and high variability in infection assays. The efforts to establish alternative HBV infection models like the use of primary tupaia hepatocytes are promising, but tupaias are until now only available to very few laboratories worldwide. Infection studies are possible with the woodchuck model but a severe disadvantage of this system is so far that recombinant WHV cannot be produced in vitro by transfection of cultured cells with cloned viral genomes. In light of the above-mentioned austerities, the DHBV model of HBV infection is a convenient and reliable system which offers several unique advantages. Most importantly, steady availability and highly reproducible infection of primary duck hepatocytes (PDHs) provide the optimal basis for in vitro and in vivo studies on the molecular and cellular biology of HBV infection under defined and controlled conditions.

Host Tropism and Species Specificity

All known hepadnaviruses are highly cell type specific and have a narrow host range restricting them to their natural host and a few closely related species. For instance, DHBV infects only certain duck and goose species but does not infect Muscovy ducks or chickens. Despite its substantial sequence homology with DHBV, HHBV does not infect ducks (see figure 1 for pedigree of avihepadnaviruses and corresponding hosts). But once the natural entry pathway is bypassed by transfection of the naked viral DNA into infection-resistant cells, replication proceeds normally. Thus, it seems that the block for efficient cross-species infection is destined at the level of viral entry. However, little is known about the viral and cellular factors involved. Although ducks and duck-derived primary hepatocytes are virtually non-permissive for HHBV, substitution of a region of the HHBV-specific preS domain by the corresponding sequence from DHBV overcomes this species barrier. As a consequence, the pseudotyped HHBV virions can efficiently infect PDHs [2]. The same applies to mammalian hepadnaviruses as shown for woolly monkey HBV pseudotyped with a small stretch of preS1 sequence from HBV, which became infectious for human hepatocytes. The so-called host-determining region (HDR) in the preS part of the avian L protein was mapped to amino acids 22–90, and an exchange of this small region also changed the species specificity [2]. These findings have largely been confirmed with an independent experimental approach by a second research group who showed that recombinant peptides containing the HDR compete with viral particles for cell binding which reduced productive infection [3]. These studies clearly indicate that the block to cross-species infection by hepadnaviruses is destined at the level of infectious viral entry and that a small domain within the preS region of the L protein plays a pivotal role in host discrimination.

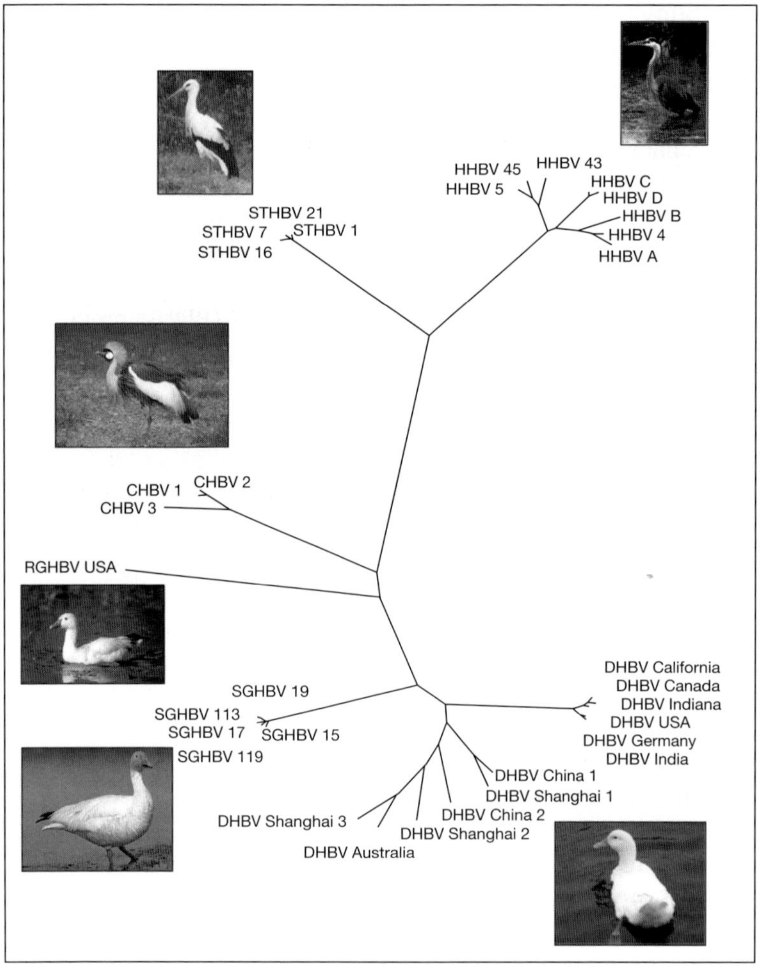

Fig. 1. Phylogenetic relationship of all known avian hepadnaviruses based on preS/S gene sequence. The corresponding natural hosts are also indicated. STHBV stands for stork HBV, HHBV for heron HBV, DHBV for duck HBV, SGHBV for snow goose HBV, RGHBV for Ross' goose HBV, and CHBV for crane HBV.

Recently, we showed that cranes are naturally infected with a novel hepadnavirus, designated CHBV [4]. Phylogenetically, cranes are very distant from ducks and are closely related to herons and storks. However, we found that CHBV infects PDHs with similar efficiency as DHBV indicating a rather broad host range of this virus at least in vitro. Whether CHBV can establish chronic infection in ducks in vivo and is as non-pathogenic as DHBV remains

Amino acids	22 37
CHBV1	Q Q L A G R M I P P M P K G T V T W S
DHBV16	N □ □ □ □ □ □ □ □ - - - □ □ □ L □ □ □
HHBV4	□ H □ □ □ □ □ □ □ □ E F S □ □ I □ T A
RGHBV	□ □ □ □ □ □ □ □ □ - - - □ □ □ □ □ □ □
SGHBV1-13	□ □ □ □ □ □ □ □ □ - - - □ G □ □ □ □ □
STHBV1	□ □ □ □ □ □ □ □ □ R E F Q □ P I □ T A

Fig. 2. Amino acid sequence alignment of part of the HDR of all five known avian hepadnaviruses. Only divergent amino acids are indicated. Hyphens mark deletions introduced for optimal alignments, squares stand for identical amino acids.

to be elucidated. Interestingly, comparison between the HDR of DHBV and the HDR of CHBV reveals a short insert of 3 amino acids (PMP) in the CHBV preS protein, a sequence similar but not identical to the analogous region of HHBV and STHBV (stork HBV), whereas all other known duck and goose hepadnaviruses have no such insert (fig. 2). It remains to be shown which sequence features of the preS protein are responsible for the unusual broad host range of CHBV and at which level of infection the block in cross-species infection is determined.

Host Cell Tropism and Determinants of Viral Infection

Infectious Entry

Infections by animal viruses begin with the attachment to their host cells followed by internalization, uncoating and delivery of the viral genome to its replication site. While factors involved in these early and most vulnerable steps of the viral life cycle have been identified for a number of viruses, little is known for hepadnaviruses [for a review, see 1 and references therein]. Hepadnaviruses replicate predominantly in hepatocytes. This marked hepatotropism seems to be mainly determined at the level of viral entry, since hepatoma cell lines, which are competent for HBV DNA replication after transfection, are not permissive for infection [5]. The tissue specificity of hepadnaviruses and the resistance of cell lines to viral infection are generally believed to be due to the absence of a selective viral receptor on the surface of these cells suggesting that the receptor is a major determinant for efficient infection. DHBV and HBV show a similar tissue tropism indicating conserved receptor(s) usage and/or entry pathways. Thus, identification of the DHBV receptor may also reveal the receptor molecule of HBV or provide a hint for a related molecule. Concerning the nature of the receptor protein for HBV, a number of cellular proteins have been described, however none of these proteins render infection-resistant cell lines or primary cells susceptible for HBV infection [6, 7]. Progress in this field has been reported recently only for the DHBV system. Two research groups have isolated a novel carboxypeptidase (CPD, also designated gp180) and proposed it to be a potential DHBV receptor [8, 9]. CPD was shown to bind both viral particles and recombinant preS protein with high affinity [10]. These findings have been confirmed and extended by showing that heterologous expression of CPD leads to efficient internalization of viral particles in resistant hepatoma cells, but not to productive infection [11]. However, the role of CPD as a DHBV receptor is complicated by the fact that heterologous expression of this protein cannot overcome the resistance of hepatoma cells to viral infection. This suggests that either additional factors are required for the establishment of a productive infection or that this molecule is not at all part of the receptor complex. Notably, the preS polypeptide of HHBV binds to duck CPD at least as strongly as the DHBV preS polypeptide [10], which implies that this cellular molecule cannot be the sole decisive determinant for viral host specificity. Further studies are clearly warranted to demonstrate whether CPD-preS binding eventually in concert with other specific steps and factors at the cellular membrane is involved in or determine together host specificity. Note also, CPD is widely expressed in several tissues, so its expression pattern does not explain the hepatotropism of DHBV. These facts indicate that CPD is not the main determinant for viral binding and uptake into the host cell, while it may still be part of a receptor complex, which mediates these steps. Consistent with this notion is the possibility that events subsequent to viral binding and internalization may determine the host range. In summary, functional receptors have not been identified for any of the hepadnaviruses and their specific role in determining tissue tropism and host range therefore remains unknown.

While attempting to identify these molecules, we have recently characterized the attachment and entry kinetics of DHBV in permissive primary hepatocytes and resistant cell lines. Therefore, we established a sensitive assay which allows for the first time to monitor virus binding and uptake in a semiquantitative manner using PCR. This binding assay revealed that in our system only a small proportion of the inoculum binds to hepatocytes. We detected only unspecific DHBV binding to the chicken cell line LMH known to be resistant to DHBV infection as evident by our failure to prevent this binding with neutralizing antisera directed against the viral preS protein. These results suggest that the attachment which we measure is specific for cells that are permissive for DHBV infection [pers. unpubl. data]. Further evidence for this conclusion was obtained by neutralization assays using suramin or neutralizing antibodies,

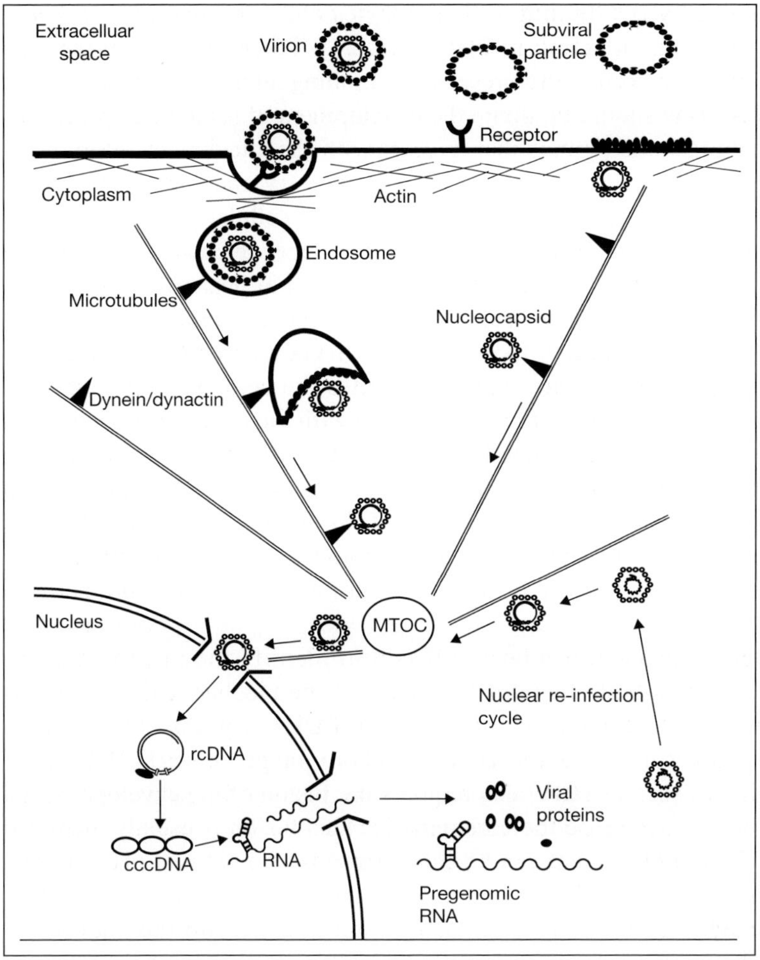

Fig. 3. Model for entry and intracellular trafficking of DHBV. The hepadnaviral life cycle starts with the attachment of virions to specific binding sites on the surface of hepatocytes mediated by the preS region of the large viral envelope protein. Following internalization and fusion of viral and cellular membranes at the plasma membrane or in endosomes, cores are released into the cytosol. The incoming viral genomes are delivered by a dynein-mediated retrograde transport along MTs to the microtubule-organizing center (MTOC) and subsequently to the nucleus. Upon its arrival in the nucleus the viral genome, the rcDNA, is converted into cccDNA (covalently closed DNA) to complete the infectious entry. All transcripts function as mRNAs and the longest of them, the pregenomic RNA, encodes for core and pol proteins. The pregenomic transcript is encapsidated together with pol into nucleocapsids and reverse transcribed into partially double-stranded DNA. These capsids are either re-transported into the nucleus, presumably by using MTs, or they are enveloped after their interaction with surface proteins in a post-ER compartment.

which all reduced virus binding to hepatocytes and subsequently markedly decreased productive infection in PDHs [23, 24]. Taken together, these data imply that our assay detects the presence of binding sites relevant for DHBV infection. This assay should facilitate the development of screening procedures to select for therapeutic ligands that interact with the attachment receptor for hepadnaviruses and thereby block viral binding, entry and subsequent infection. It could also lead to identification of viral and cellular partners involved in specific binding of the virus to the host cell surface which should then shed light on the determinants of species and liver tropism of hepadnaviruses.

To establish infection, the virus does not only have to bind specifically to its primary receptor, but also to enter the cell via a selective pathway. To determine the amount of virus which penetrates the cellular membrane in a given time, we used a protease protection assay with the assumption that internalized virus should be protected from an externally active protease. We observed that 1 h after attachment about 70% of bound DHBV was taken up and internalization was complete within 3 h [23]. In summary, our data show that only a limited amount of DHBV virions specifically binds to hepatocytes, but that these viruses are very efficiently internalized via a yet unidentified pathway.

For several reasons it has been difficult to identify the infectious entry pathway of HBVs on both the ultrastructural and the biochemical level. It has been shown that infectious entry of DHBV in PDHs requires energy which implicates the advocation of active cellular and/or viral processes [12]. Entry of enveloped viruses such as HBV also requires the fusion of the envelope with a cellular membrane to release the core particle. This fusion is usually mediated by viral envelope proteins and can be categorized by the optimal pH required. Viruses which enter the cell in a pH-independent manner usually fuse either with the plasma membrane or after being internalized with the endosomal membranes. In contrast, viruses that enter the cell in a low pH-dependent manner fuse only after internalization and exposure to an acidic environment. Currently, only indirect evidence is available for the postulated fusion event of HBV. Studies addressing the pH dependency of viral entry in the DHBV model led to conflicting conclusions [12–14]. However, the weight of data suggests an entry route which does not require passage through a highly acidic compartment. Irrespective of the mechanism of virus entry, core particles have to deliver their cargo, the viral genome, into the nucleus where the first event in viral replication accessible to experimental investigation is the conversion of the incoming viral rcDNA (relaxed circular) genomes to cccDNA (covalently closed circular). Since the latter serves as a pivotal template for the transcription of all viral messages, its formation indicates initiation of a productive infection [15, 16]. Conversion of rc- into cccDNA in liver cells is detectable within the first 24 h after virus inoculation. Thus, after the efficient viral uptake there is an unusually long gap of 13–17 h before the appearance of nuclear viral cccDNA indicating successful entry and infection. This gap suggests that there is a rate-limiting post-entry step either preceding cccDNA formation which involves viral uncoating and nuclear genome transport or required for rc- to cccDNA conversion.

Intracellular Trafficking

Viruses not only depend on the host machinery for internalization but also for their trafficking within the cytoplasm and the ability to find the correct site for replication. Such trafficking depends on specific post-internalization membrane sorting and, in some cases, direct interactions of viral particles with the cytoskeleton [17]. Several lines of experiments support the assertion that components of the cytoskeleton are essential host co-factors for viral replication [for reviews, see 18, 19]. Upon entry, viruses use the host cytoskeleton to move within the cell towards their respective replication center as known for adenovirus, herpes simplex virus (HSV) and HIV [for review, see 20]. Thus, after attachment to a hepatocyte, a highly polarized epithelial cell type, a series of tightly coordinated and directional steps is presumably required for hepadnaviral transport through the cytoplasm before the viral genome is successfully delivered to the nucleus. To test the potential requirement of the cytoskeleton for intracellular trafficking of incoming hepadnaviral particles, we used drugs which inactivate the actin or the microtubule network. Disruption of actin fibers did not interfere with infection, it even increased the number of attached virions on the cell surface and resulted in enhancement of viral infection [23]. This implicates that the actin cortex is dispensable for infection and may even pose a steric hindrance during viral entry. In contrast, treatment of the cells with microtubule-disrupting drugs resulted in abrogation of infection, cccDNA formation and amplification [23]. We excluded that this effect was due to a lack of viral binding and internalization into the host cells. Moreover, overexpression of dynamitin, a co-factor subunit of the motor protein complex dynactin-dynein, which mediates transport along microtubules (MTs), also reduced DHBV infection presumably by disruption of this complex [pers. unpublished data]. The data available so far indicate that MTs play a critical role in a transport step occurring after virus attachment and internalization and prior to the core-mediated delivery of incoming viral genomes into the nucleus. Thus, internalization by the native entry pathway of the virus is necessary, but not sufficient to establish a successful infection (see figure 3 for our current model of DHBV infection). Disruption of the MTs during virus trafficking presumably irreversibly blocks progression of virions to cellular compartment(s) where fusion can occur. The incoming viral particles might then be arrested and targeted for degradation. In line with this notion is the proposal that MT-mediated transport is part of the innate cellular antiviral response through delivery of abnormal cargo to aggreasomes for proteolytic clearance [21]. Further evidence supporting this scenario is provided by the fact that certain protease inhibitors enhance HIV infection [22].

The infectious entry pathway of hepadnaviruses appears to involve a series of highly coordinated and directional steps leading to the nuclear delivery of viral genomes essential for the establishment of a productive infection. These steps may, alone or in combination, determine the strict species and host cell tropism common to all hepadnaviruses.

Acknowledgments

The HPI is supported by the Freie und Hansestadt Hamburg and the Bundesministerium für Gesundheit und Soziale Sicherung. This work was supported by grants from the BMBF (Hepnet and NGFN). L.L. is recipient of a DAAD scholarship.

References

1 Ganem D, Schneider RJ: Hepadnaviridae: The viruses and their replication; in Knipe DM, Howley PM (eds): Fields Virology. Philadelphia, Lippincott Williams & Wilkins, 2002, pp 2923–2969.

2 Ishikawa T, Ganem D: The pre-S domain of the large viral envelope protein determines host range in avian hepatitis B viruses. Proc Natl Acad Sci USA 1995;92:6259–6263.

3 Urban S, Breiner KM, Fehler F, Klingmuller U, Schaller H: Avian hepatitis B virus infection is initiated by the interaction of a distinct pre-S subdomain with the cellular receptor gp180. J Virol 1998;72:8089–8097.

4 Prassolov A, Hohenberg H, Kalinina T, Schneider C, Cova L, Krone O, Frolich K, Will H, Sirma H: New hepatitis B virus of cranes that has an unexpected broad host range. J Virol 2003;77:1964–1976.

5 Hirsch R, Colgrove R, Ganem D: Replication of duck hepatitis B virus in two differentiated human hepatoma cell lines after transfection with cloned viral DNA. Virology 1988;167:136–142.

6 De Falco S, Ruvoletto MG, Verdoliva A, Ruvo M, Raucci A, Marino M, Senatore S, Cassani G, Alberti A, Pontisso P, Fassina G: Cloning and expression of a novel hepatitis B virus-binding protein from HepG2 cells. J Biol Chem 2001;276:36613–36623.

7 Neurath AR, Strick N, Li YY: Cells transfected with human interleukin-6 cDNA acquire binding sites for the hepatitis B virus envelope protein. J Exp Med 1992;176:1561–1569.

8 Kuroki K, Cheung R, Marion PL, Ganem D: A cell surface protein that binds avian hepatitis B virus particles. J Virol 1994;68:2091–2096.

9 Tong S, Li J, Wands JR: Interaction between duck hepatitis B virus and a 170-kilodalton cellular protein is mediated through a neutralizing epitope of the pre-S region and occurs during viral infection. J Virol 1995;69:7106–7112.

10 Urban S, Schwarz C, Marx UC, Zentgraf H, Schaller H, Multhaup G: Receptor recognition by a hepatitis B virus reveals a novel mode of high affinity virus-receptor interaction. EMBO J 2000;19:1217–1227.

11 Breiner KM, Urban S, Schaller H: Carboxypeptidase D (gp180), a Golgi-resident protein, functions in the attachment and entry of avian hepatitis B viruses. J Virol 1998;72:8098–8104.

12 Kock J, Borst EM, Schlicht HJ: Uptake of duck hepatitis B virus into hepatocytes occurs by endocytosis but does not require passage of the virus through an acidic intracellular compartment. J Virol 1996;70:5827–5831.
13 Offensperger WB, Offensperger S, Walter E, Blum HE, Gerok W: Inhibition of duck hepatitis B virus infection by lysosomotropic agents. Virology 1991;183:415–418.
14 Rigg RJ, Schaller H: Duck hepatitis B virus infection of hepatocytes is not dependent on low pH. J Virol 1992;66:2829–2836.
15 Kock J, Schlicht HJ: Analysis of the earliest steps of hepadnavirus replication: Genome repair after infectious entry into hepatocytes does not depend on viral polymerase activity. J Virol 1993;67:4867–4874.
16 Weiser B, Ganem D, Seeger C, Varmus HE: Closed circular viral DNA and asymmetrical heterogeneous forms in livers from animals infected with ground squirrel hepatitis virus. J Virol 1983;48:1–9.
17 Smith GA, Enquist LW: Break ins and break outs: Viral interactions with the cytoskeleton of mammalian cells. Annu Rev Cell Dev Biol 2002;18:135–161.
18 Sodeik B: Mechanisms of viral transport in the cytoplasm. Trends Microbiol 2000;8:465–472.
19 Ploubidou A, Way M: Viral transport and the cytoskeleton. Curr Opin Cell Biol 2001;13:97–105.
20 Luftig RB, Holleran EA, Karki S, Holzbaur EL: Does the cytoskeleton play a significant role in animal virus replication? J Theor Biol 1982;99:173–191.
21 Sodeik B: Unchain my heart, baby let me go – the entry and intracellular transport of HIV. J Cell Biol 2002;159:393–395.
22 Schwartz O, Marechal V, Friguet B, Arenzana-Seisdedos F, Heard JM: Antiviral activity of the proteasome on incoming human immunodeficiency virus type 1. J Virol 1998;72:3845–3850.
23 Funk A, Mhamdi M, Lin L, Will H, Sirma H: Itinerary of hepatitis B viruses: delineation of restriction points critical for infectious entry. J Virol 2004;78(15):8289–8300.
24 Funk A, Hohenberg H, Mhamdi H, Will H, Sirma H: Spread of hepatitis B viruses in vitro requires extracellular progeny and may be codetermined by polarized egress. J Virol 2004;78(8): 3977–3983.

Hüseyin Sirma
Department of General Virology, Heinrich-Pette-Institut für experimentelle Virologie und Immunologie an der Universität Hamburg
Postfach 201652, DE–20206 Hamburg (Germany)
Tel. +49 40 4805 1226; Fax +49 40 4805 1222, E-Mail sirma@hpi.uni-hamburg.de

von Weizsäcker F, Roggendorf M (eds): Models of Viral Hepatitis.
Monogr Virol. Basel, Karger, 2005, vol 25, pp 66–80

T-Cell Response to Hepatitis B and C Virus: Lessons from the Chimpanzee Model

R. Thimme[a,c], *J. Bukh*[b], *H.C. Spangenberg*[c], *S.F. Wieland*[a], *H.E. Blum*[c], *R.H. Purcell*[b], *F.V. Chisari*[a]

[a]Department of Molecular and Experimental Medicine, The Scripps Research Institute, La Jolla, Calif., USA; [b]Hepatitis Viruses Section, Laboratory of Infectious Diseases, National Institutes of Health, Bethesda, Md., USA, and [c]Department of Medicine II, University of Freiburg, Germany

Several studies in acutely and chronically infected patients have led to the conclusion that the cellular immune response is responsible for viral clearance and disease pathogenesis during hepatitis B virus (HBV) and hepatitis C virus (HCV) infection. However, several important aspects of hepatitis B and C immunobiology can not be defined in infected patients. For example, the kinetics, quality and vigor of the early antiviral T-cell response soon after exposure to these viruses are likely to determine the outcome of infection. These parameters are not testable in humans who acquire the infection several weeks or months prior to the onset of clinically apparent disease. Furthermore, since for ethical reasons no liver biopsies can be obtained during the acute phase of liver disease, there is no information about the host-virus interactions at the site of disease, the liver. In addition, depletion experiments of T-cell subtypes that may help to define the role of each T-cell subpopulation (e.g. $CD4^+$ and $CD8^+$ cells) can not be performed in humans. For these reasons, several investigators have studied the T-cell response to HBV and HCV in the chimpanzee model, the only animal model available for the study of the immune response during the natural course of HBV and HCV infection. This review will summarize recent findings about the role of virus-specific T-cell responses during acute and chronic HBV and

HCV infection that have been forthcoming from studies in experimentally infected chimpanzees.

Hepatitis B Virus

T-Cell Response to HBV in Humans

Several studies have shown that the peripheral blood cytotoxic T lymphocyte (CTL) response to HBV is polyclonal and multispecific in patients with acute viral hepatitis and persists indefinitely after recovery, when it is maintained by continued antigenic stimulation by residual virus that persists, apparently harmlessly, in healthy convalescent individuals [1–5]. In contrast, the CTL response to HBV is relatively weak in patients with chronic HBV infection, except during spontaneous disease flares or interferon (IFN)-induced recovery, when it is readily detectable [5].

Studies in the HBV transgenic mouse model revealed that, in addition to causing viral hepatitis, virus-specific T cells as well as NK and NKT cells can abolish HBV expression and replication without killing the hepatocytes and that this antiviral activity is mediated by interferon-γ (IFN-γ) and tumor necrosis factor-α [6, 7].

The studies performed in acutely infected humans and in transgenic mice have added further important information about the nature of the T-cell response to HBV. However, several important questions have remained due to the limitations of both models. For example, the kinetics, quality and vigor of the early antiviral T-cell response soon after exposure to these viruses and the intrahepatic T-cell response can not be easily studied in humans. The early host-virus interactions can also not be studied in transgenic mice that are not infected by the virus. However, they can be studied in susceptible animal models, such as chimpanzees. Chimpanzees are ideal for the analysis of the early immune events in the blood and liver of acute HBV infection since they are the only species other than humans that can be infected by HBV [8]. Indeed, after inoculation with infectious sera, chimpanzees develop typical cases of acute self-limited HBV infection characterized by transient HBs and HBe antigenemia, biochemical and histological evidence of viral hepatitis, antibody seroconversion, and clearance of viral antigens and HBV DNA.

In order to define the early host-virus interactions during acute HBV infection, we studied the early virological and immunological events in acutely infected chimpanzees. In addition, depletion experiments of $CD4^+$ and $CD8^+$ T cells were performed to examine the extent to which each T-cell subset contributes to the control of acute HBV infection. All the results described in the following were performed in the laboratory of Prof. Frank Chisari, Scripps Research Institute, La Jolla, Calif., USA.

Viral Clearance without Destruction of Infected Cells during Acute HBV Infection

A comprehensive analysis of the virological, histological and immunological intrahepatic events during acute HBV infection was performed in 2 chimpanzees that were inoculated with 1×10^8 genome equivalents of a cloned isolate of HBV (ayw subtype) from the serum of HBV transgenic mice that replicate the virus at high titers. Both chimpanzees developed typical cases of acute, self-limited viral hepatitis [9]. Importantly, at least 90% of the viral DNA was eliminated from the liver during acute HBV infection by non-cytolytic processes that preceded and were independent of the immune elimination of infected hepatocytes. Indeed, viral replication was almost completely abolished several weeks before the peak of T-cell infiltration and liver disease. The disappearance of HBV DNA occurred soon after CD3 and inflammatory cytokines, especially IFN-γ appeared in the liver [9]. Importantly, as has been described above, IFN-γ also inhibits HBV gene expression and replication in the liver of transgenic mice [7]. These results demonstrated for the first time that a non-cytopathic control of HBV replication (probably mediated by IFN-γ) might also contribute to viral clearance during natural HBV infection.

Overlap of Class 1 and CTL Repertoires between Humans and Chimpanzees

In a follow-up study, protocols were established to study the virus-specific T-cell response in the same 2 acutely infected chimpanzees. Using an in vitro peptide stimulation strategy, it was shown that both animals produced peripheral blood CTL responses to several HBV-encoded epitopes [10] that are known to be recognized by HLA-class I restricted CTL in acutely infected humans [10]. The peptides recognized by each animal corresponded with the ability of its PATR class I molecules to bind peptides containing the HLA-A2 and HLA-B7 supermotifs [10]. In sum, these results demonstrated that the CTL repertoire overlaps in humans and chimpanzees. They also showed the feasibility of using chimpanzees to elucidate the CTL response to HBV, thereby offering the opportunity to study the very early virus-specific T-cell response in the blood and liver in additional prospective studies.

Analysis of a Successful Immune Response against HBV

By using the newly developed protocols, the peripheral and intrahepatic HBV-specific T-cell responses were monitored in a chimpanzee that was used as a control animal for depletion studies described below. The animal was inoculated with high titer transgenic mouse serum (1×10^8 genome equivalents) that has been shown to cause a typical course of acute HBV infection in chimpanzees (see above). Blood and liver biopsies were obtained at weekly intervals after infection and tested for virological, immunological and histological parameters. As shown in figure 1A, HBV DNA was first detectable in the liver 5 weeks after inoculation and peaked at week 8 [11]. Between weeks 8 and 11, the HBV DNA content of the liver abruptly deceased by more than 95%. The reduction of viral DNA corresponded with the appearance and persistence of IFN-γ expression in the liver. In this phase of infection, sALT levels were only slightly elevated. These results again strongly suggest that the initial phase of viral clearance may reflect primarily non-cytopathic inhibition of viral replication by cytokines, such as IFN-γ. The peak of sALT activity was reached by week 14 and coincided with the final elimination of HBV DNA. Thus, this prolonged episode of liver disease may reflect the destructive potential of the immune response which appears to be required for the final elimination of the virus.

Importantly, HBV-specific $CD4^+$ and $CD8^+$ T-cell responses were first detectable in the blood 2–3 weeks after inoculation (data not shown). As shown in figure 1A, intrahepatic HBcAg-specific $CD4^+$ T-cell responses were first detectable in week 6 and surged by week 10 to levels that were sustained for the rest of the study. HBV-specific $CD8^+$ T-cell responses became first detectable in the liver in week 10 coinciding with the appearance of CD3 and IFN-γ mRNA in the liver [11]. Importantly, the onset of the virus-specific $CD8^+$ T-cell response correlated with the first rapid reduction in HBV DNA and the onset of mild liver disease. The results of this study suggest that virus-specific $CD4^+$ and $CD8^+$ T cells are primed early in the infection but do not enter the liver until a few weeks later when especially $CD8^+$ T cells are temporally associated with liver disease and the final elimination of the virus. The important role of the adaptive immune response is also supported by a genomic analysis of the host response to HBV in the liver [12]. Interestingly, HBV did not induce genes during entry and expansion, suggesting that HBV is a stealth virus early in the infection. In contrast, a large number of T-cell-derived IFN-γ-regulated genes were induced during viral clearance, reflecting the impact of an adaptive T-cell response that inhibits viral replication and kills infected cells, thereby terminating viral infection.

$CD8^+$ T Cells but not $CD4^+$ T Cells Mediate Viral Clearance and Disease Pathogenesis during Acute HBV Infection

Although the $CD4^+$ and $CD8^+$ T-cell responses to HBV are thought to be crucial for the control of HBV infection, the relative contribution of each T-cell subset as an effector of viral clearance was not known. To examine this question, we monitored the course of HBV infection in a $CD4^+$-depleted (fig. 1B) and a $CD8^+$-depleted (fig. 1C) chimpanzee. These 2 animals were inoculated with high titer HBV DNA positive transgenic mouse serum and at the expected time of onset of viremia, the animals were treated with monoclonal antibodies to human CD4 or CD8 [11] that have been previously shown to specifically deplete $CD4^+$ and $CD8^+$

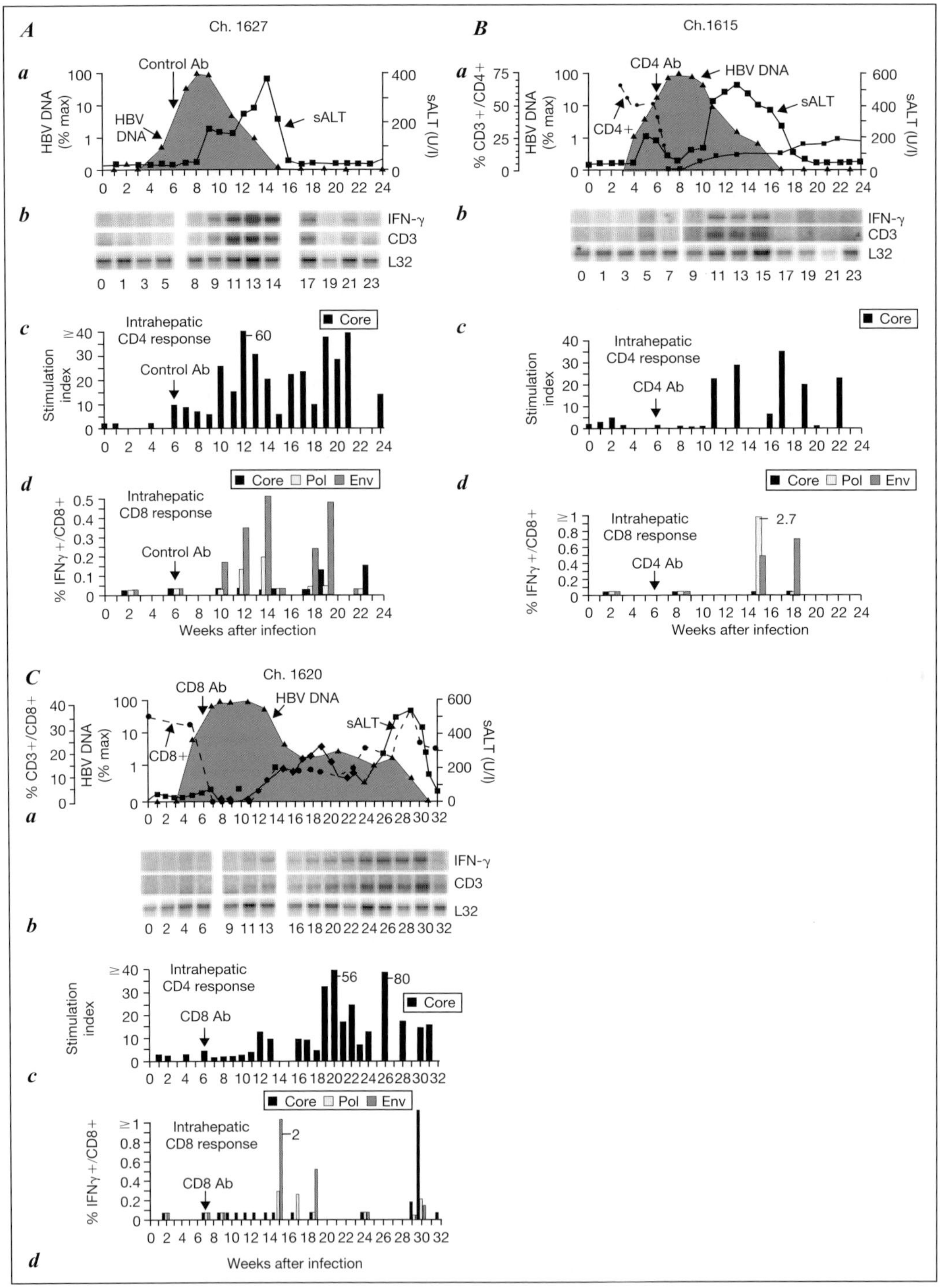
A
Ch. 1627
B
Ch.1615
Control Ab
HBV DNA
sALT
IFN-γ
CD3
L32
Intrahepatic CD4 response
Stimulation index
Core
Pol
Env
Intrahepatic CD8 response
% IFNγ+/CD8+
Weeks after infection
CD4 Ab
CD4+
% CD3+/CD4+
HBV DNA (% max)
sALT (U/l)
C
Ch. 1620
CD8 Ab
CD8+
% CD3+/CD8+

T cells in macaques and chimpanzees [13, 14]. As compared to the control animal, the resolution of infection was slightly delayed in the CD4-depleted animal, presumably reflecting the delayed accumulation of HBV-specific $CD4^+$ and $CD8^+$ T cells in the liver (fig. 1B). This was probably due to the effect of anti-CD4 antibody on the total circulating $CD4^+$ T-cell count. However, although CD4 depletion appeared to slightly modulate the duration of infection in this animal, it is likely that they are not the principal effectors of viral clearance and disease pathogenesis in HBV infection. In contrast to the minor effects observed during CD4 depletion, CD8 depletion greatly prolonged the infection and delayed the onset of viral clearance and liver disease until $CD8^+$ T cells reappeared in the circulation and virus-specific $CD8^+$ T cells entered the liver (fig. 1C) [11]. Indeed, in the absence of $CD8^+$ cells, the duration of peak infection was prolonged and the onset of the initial rapid decrease in HBV DNA levels and increase in serum ALT activity was delayed. In addition, the time required for both the first phase of viral clearance and for the final elimination of the virus was markedly delayed and prolonged in the CD8-depleted animal. It is important to note that the reappearance of $CD8^+$ cells correlated with the appearance of IFN-γ producing virus-specific $CD8^+$ T cells in the liver, the onset of a mild liver disease, the appearance of IFN-γ mRNA in the liver and a 50-fold reduction in total liver HBV DNA (fig. 1C). These results suggest that HBV replication is inhibited early non-cytopathically by a CD8-dependent and probably IFN-γ-associated manner. The final elimination of the virus occurred several months later and was associated with a rebound of $CD8^+$ cells to baseline levels, a surge of the intrahepatic $CD8^+$ T-cell response, a surge in intrahepatic IFN-γ mRNA and a surge in sALT activity (fig. 1C). Thus, our results demonstrate that intrahepatic HBV-specific $CD8^+$ T cells are required for rapid viral clearance during acute HBV infection. In addition, the data suggest the existence of dual antiviral functions that overlap temporally during natural infection but can be clearly separated by CD8 depletion: a primarily non-cytolytic

Fig. 1. Course of acute HBV infection in chimpanzees after experimental inoculation with HBV in the presence or absence of $CD4^+$ and $CD8^+$ cells. All animals were inoculated intravenously with high titer HBV-positive transgenic mouse serum. Ch.1627 was injected with an irrelevant control antibody (***A***). Ch.1615 was injected with a CD4-specific monoclonal antibody (***B***) and Ch.1620 was injected with a CD8-specific monoclonal antibody (***C***). Intrahepatic HBV DNA is expressed as the percentage (% max) of the corresponding peak HBV DNA levels in the liver of each animal. ***b*** Total RNA analyzed from the liver was analyzed for the intrahepatic expression of CD3, IFN-γ and L32 by an RNAse protection assay. ***c*** The intrahepatic $CD4^+$ T-cell response to HBcAg is expressed as the SI. ***d*** Intrahepatic $CD8^+$ T-cell responses are expressed as the percentage of intrahepatic $CD8^+$ T cells that produce IFN-γ after stimulation with autologous EBV B cells that were infected with recombinant vaccinia viruses expressing the HBV core, polymerase and large envelope protein after subtraction of their responsiveness to the same B cells infected by wild-type vaccinia viruses. The vertical arrows indicate antibody treatments.

CD8$^+$-dependent mechanism that may be mediated by IFN-γ and a primarily cytolytic mechanism that clears the remaining infected cells.

Hepatitis C Virus

T-Cell Response to HCV in Humans

There is a growing consensus that the development of a relatively strong CD4$^+$ and CD8$^+$ T-cell response to HCV correlates with the resolution of the infection [11, 15–18]. However, the early virological and immunological determinants of HCV clearance, persistence and disease are not well defined, because most acutely infected patients have not been studied until after the onset of liver disease. One study has recently described the virological and immunological features of acute HCV infection in 5 healthcare workers after accidental needlestick inoculation [19]. It was found that viremia was first detectable several weeks before the appearance of virus-specific T cells in the blood, that viral hepatitis coincided with the onset of a peripheral T-cell response, that viral clearance was temporally associated with the production of IFN-γ by CD8$^+$ cells, and that it was not accompanied by a surge in liver disease. In contrast, chronic infection developed in 2 asymptomatic subjects who failed to produce a significant T-cell response and in 2 symptomatic patients who initially mounted strong T-cell responses that ultimately waned [19].

For ethical reasons, liver biopsies were not performed in these patients, so the virus-host interactions at the site of infection could not be studied. In addition, very little information has been available about the relationship between the kinetics of viral spread and the induction of the intrahepatic T-cell response to HCV, the efficiency with which T cells home to the liver, how long they survive or how well they function once they arrive. In addition, the role of virus-induced or T-cell-derived cytokines in viral clearance has not been defined. To address these important issues, we and others have studied the immune response in acutely infected chimpanzees.

Courses of Acute HCV Infection in Chimpanzees

Currently, the only animal model for HCV infection is the chimpanzee. Hepatitis C (or non-A, non-B) was first transmitted to chimpanzees more than 20 years ago. Numerous studies since then have detailed the course of HCV infection in chimpanzees and it has been shown that the course of infection in chimpanzees is similar in its diversity to that in humans [20]. In general, acute experimental HCV infection is characterized by early appearance of viremia within a few days after infection and peak viral titers of 10^5–10^7 GE/ml between weeks 7 and 12. Most animals have evidence of hepatitis with elevated sALT levels and necro-inflammatory changes in liver biopsies. Some chimpanzees resolve the infection but most progress to chronic infection [20].

We have recently described three different courses of HCV infection in acutely infected chimpanzees: sustained viral clearance, transient viral clearance followed by persistence and chronic infection that persisted at initial peak titers [19]. Irrespective of the course of infection, viral RNA became detectable within 1 week in all animals and viral titers rose several orders of magnitude very rapidly after their initial appearance (fig. 2). In animals that displayed sustained viral clearance, rapid viral decreases were observed between weeks 9 and 11. The rapid viral decrease was associated in 1 animal with a surge of liver disease whereas viral clearance occurred in another animal in the absence of any elevation of sALT activity. Animals with transient viral clearance also displayed early peak viral titers that rapidly decreased by 3–4 orders of magnitude to become undetectable. However, the virus became detectable again and it fluctuated thereafter between undetectable and $10^{3.8}$ GE/ml, indicating low level persistent infection. Two animals developed viral persistence with viral titers persisting at initial peak titers (fig. 2).

Analysis of Successful Immune Responses against HCV

Cooper et al. [21] first described successful immune responses against HCV in acutely infected chimpanzees. They showed that 2 (previously vaccinated) animals that terminated infection made strong intrahepatic CTL responses but poor antibody responses. In both resolving animals, virus-specific CTL targeted at least six different viral regions. Interestingly, these HCV-specific T cells persisted in the liver tissue of these animals for more than 1 year after resolution. In contrast, animals progressing to chronic hepatitis generated weaker CTL responses in the acute phase of infection [21]. To define the role of the peripheral versus the intrahepatic HCV-specific T-cell response, the relationship between the kinetics of viral spread and the induction of the intrahepatic T-cell response and the role of T-cell-derived cytokines, we analyzed the HCV-specific T-cell response and intrahepatic cytokine profiles in 6 acutely infected animals [19]. These studies revealed several new important aspects of the host virus relationship during acute HCV infection. First, HCV spread is so rapid that it outpaces the induction of a cellular immune response by several weeks. Second, HCV is a strong inducer of type I IFN but it is relatively resistant to its antiviral activity. Third, the intrahepatic virus-specific $CD4^+$ and $CD8^+$ T-cell response correlates with the control of the infection, whereas the peripheral T-cell response does not. Fourth, major decreases in viral titer in animals that permanently or transiently clear the virus are accompanied by early, vigorous and multispecific, IFN-γ producing intrahepatic $CD4^+$ and $CD8^+$ T-cell responses. Fifth, relatively stable viral titers occur in the absence of an intrahepatic virus-specific T-cell response or IFN-γ. In addition, these results

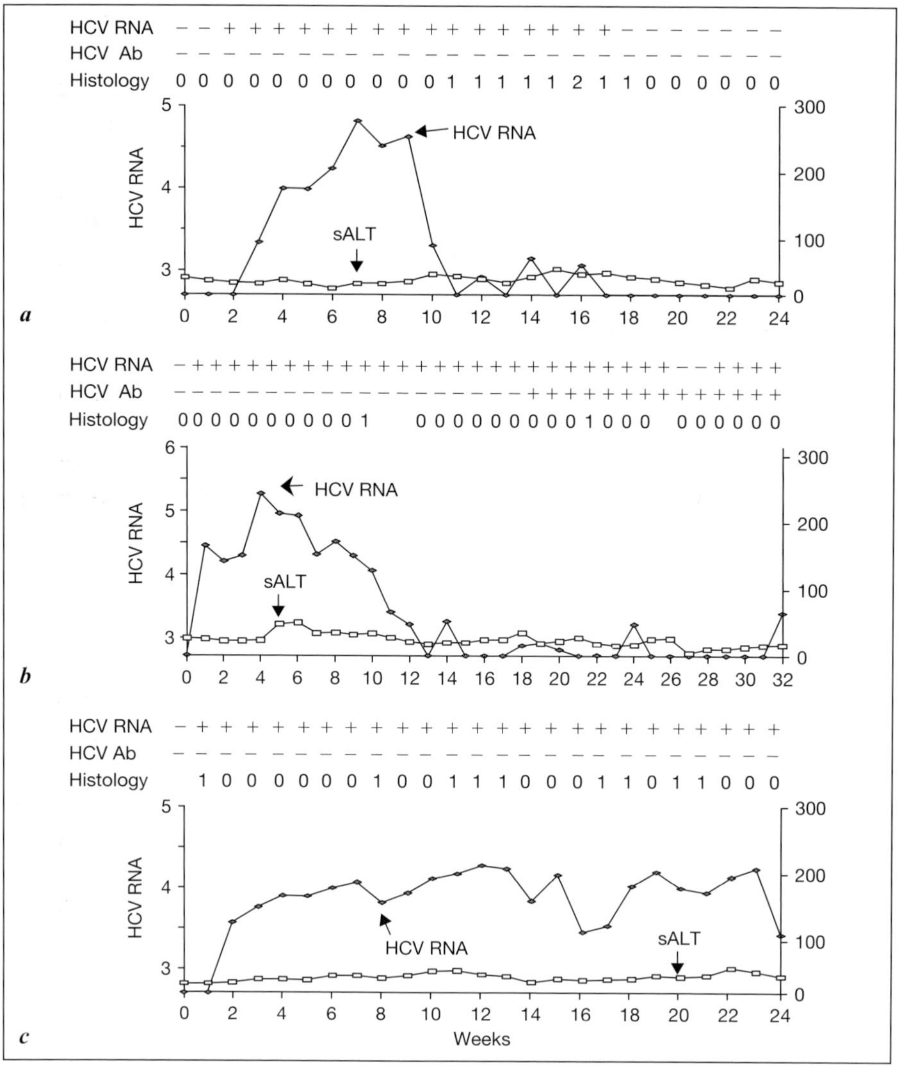

Fig. 2. Three different courses of HCV infection in acute HCV infection: (***a***) sustained viral clearance, (***b***) transient viral clearance followed by (***c***) persistence and chronic infection that persisted at initial peak titers. Quantitative HCV RNA levels were expressed as log GEs per millimeter of serum. HCV RNA was also monitored by in-house RT-nested PCR and results are indicated as + or –. ALT activity was expressed as units per liter. HCV antibody responses reflect the results of an HCV EIA-2 assay. Liver biopsies were examined for necroinflammatory changes.

also suggest that the control of infection can also occur in the absence of biochemical evidence of liver disease, suggesting the involvement of non-cytolytic T-cell effector functions as we have described above for HBV.

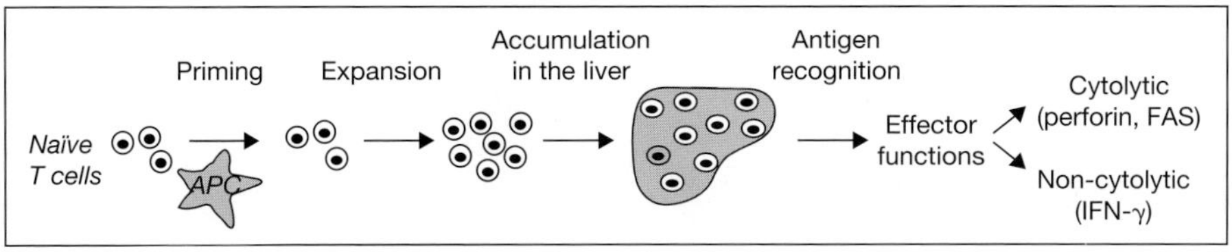

Fig. 3. Role of virus-specific T cells in the control of acute HCV infection. After priming, HCV-specific T cells expand, accumulate in the infected liver and perform different antiviral effector functions.

The single most important observation from our study was that rapid control of acute HCV infection is associated with a vigorous intrahepatic $CD4^+$ and $CD8^+$ T-cell response [19]. The key event is the accumulation of T cells in the liver not their induction in the periphery. However, the mechanisms used by the intrahepatic T cells to eliminate or control the infection remain to be determined. It is important to note that viral clearance could occur in absence of liver disease, suggesting that non-cytolytic effector functions were operative. Interestingly, IFN-γ was detectable in the liver of the animals that cleared or controlled the virus [19], raising the possibility that IFN-γ might perform antiviral effector functions during acute HCV infection, similar to its ability to control HBV replication in transgenic mice and acutely infected chimpanzees [6]. The important role of IFN-γ in viral clearance is further supported by the finding that IFN-γ, either exogenous or endogenously produced by virus-specific $CD8^+$ T cells inhibits the replication of HCV in the replicon model [22, 23]. In addition, genomic analysis of acutely infected chimpanzees revealed that transient or sustained viral clearance was associated with the up-regulation of IFN-γ-induced genes in the liver [24]. The intrahepatic induction of IFN-γ correlated well with the detection of the intrahepatic virus-specific T-cell responses, suggesting that IFN-γ is produced by T cells that accumulate in the infected organ. In sum, these studies have clearly demonstrated the important role of virus-specific T cells in the control of acute HCV infection (fig. 3). It is also important to note that another study failed to show an association between the outcome of acute HCV infection and the intrahepatic induction of T-cell or cytokine markers, peripheral T-cell responses or viral escape mutations suggesting that chimpanzees may also recover from acute HCV infection by mechanisms other than the induction of readily detectable HCV-specific T-cell responses [25].

Mechanisms of Viral Persistence during Acute HCV Infection in Chimpanzees

Studies in acutely infected chimpanzees have also revealed different mechanisms that contribute to viral persistence. Erickson et al. [26] showed

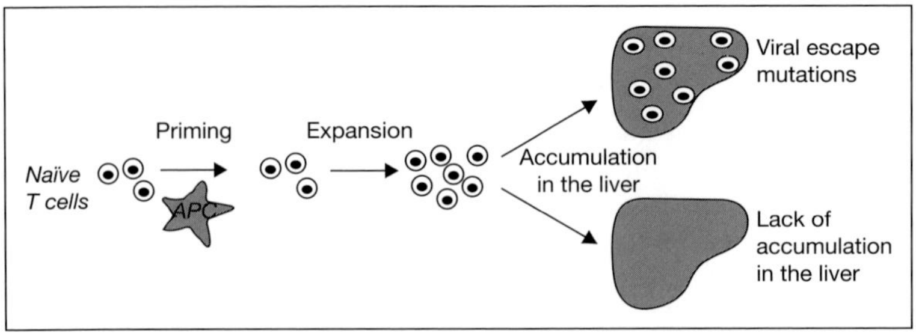

Fig. 4. Different mechanisms contribute to viral persistence during acute HCV infection in chimpanzees, such as the development of viral escape mutations or the lack of accumulation of virus-specific $CD8^+$ T cells in the liver.

that the outcome of HCV infection is predicted by escape mutations in epitopes that are targeted by virus-specific $CD8^+$ T-cell responses (fig. 4). Indeed, all chimpanzees with evolving viral persistence acquired mutations in multiple epitopes that impaired class I MHC binding and/or T-cell recognition. Most escape mutations appeared during the acute phase of infection and remained fixed in the quasispecies for years without further diversification. In contrast, animals that spontaneously resolved acute HCV infection did not develop viral escape mutations [26]. It is important to note, however, that the importance of viral escape mutations for the development of HCV persistence is still unclear. Indeed, viral escape occurs typically in the presence of a CTL response that is focused on a single viral epitope. This type of T-cell response is unusual, however, during acute HCV infection. Accordingly, the loss of a single epitope would probably not be sufficient for the survival of viral escape mutants. It is also important to emphasize that selection of escape variants occurred in the presence of an HCV-specific T-cell response that was significantly weaker compared to animals that were able to clear the virus [21, 26]. Thus, the different outcomes of infection, clearance versus persistence, may not be explained primarily by the occurrence of viral escape mutations but by initially weak virus-specific T-cell responses that make viral escape possible. Based on this concept, escape may be the result rather than the cause of viral persistence. Additional studies are needed to resolve this interesting question.

The establishment of viral escape mutations is probably not the only mechanism of T-cell failure that may lead to viral persistence. Indeed, the lack of virus-specific T cells to accumulate in the liver may also contribute to viral persistence. Indeed, animals that developed chronic infection with HCV viral titers that persisted at initial peak titers had no detectable virus-specific intrahepatic $CD8^+$ T-cell responses and no intrahepatic induction of IFN-γ. Interestingly, however, peripheral virus-specific T-cell responses became detectable in these animals, indicating that not a primary failure to induce T cells but a failure of T cells to accumulate in the liver may also contribute to the development of viral persistence [27]. The lack of T-cell accumulation in the liver can be explained either by rapid intrahepatic deletion of T cells (e.g. by activation induced cell death) or by a lack of homing of cells to the infected tissue. In sum, the studies performed in acutely infected chimpanzees suggest that HCV persistence is a multifactorial process. Clearly, additional studies are needed to identify the precise mechanisms that determine the outcome of infection in acutely infected animals.

Protective Immunity

In recent years another important question that has been evaluated in the chimpanzee model was if HCV-specific immune responses mediate sterilizing and/or protective immunity on reinfection. Earlier reports suggested that sterilizing immunity to HCV does not exist. Indeed, multiple episodes of acute HCV infection have been reported in chimpanzees [28, 29]. In these studies, 4 chimpanzees that had resolved acute HCV infection with genotype 1a or 1b strains again developed viremia when rechallenged with homologous or heterologous viruses. Interestingly, however, in most cases, the viremia was shorter following rechallenge. Nevertheless, it was concluded from these studies that HCV does not induce sterilizing or protective immunity. Recent studies in chimpanzees, however, have challenged this conclusion. Indeed, these studies demonstrated that chimpanzees that had previously recovered from HCV infection and were rechallenged with HCV showed a milder course of liver disease and achieved viral clearance within a few weeks [30–32]. Viral clearance correlated with strong peripheral memory T-cell responses and intrahepatic IFN-γ production [30–32]. The relative contribution of $CD4^+$ and $CD8^+$ T cells to protective immunity has been studied recently in chimpanzees serially infected with HCV [33, 34]. While viral clearance of a first infection took 3–4 months, viremia after a second infection was terminated within 2 weeks, matching the concept of protective immunity. Antibody-mediated depletion of $CD8^+$ T cells prior to a third infection prolonged viral replication despite presence of memory $CD4^+$ T cells. Importantly, viremia was not terminated until HCV-specific intrahepatic $CD8^+$ T cells recovered about 6 weeks after infection [33]. Antibody-mediated depletion of $CD4^+$ T cells before reinfection, however, resulted in persistent, low-level viremia despite functional intrahepatic memory $CD8^+$ T-cell responses. Importantly, the absence of $CD4^+$ T-cell help was associated with the emergence of viral escape mutations in MHC class I epitopes [34]. These data indicate that $CD8^+$ T cells are the primary effector cells mediating protective immunity. However, they also suggest that $CD4^+$ T-cell help is required for $CD8^+$ T cells to keep pace with the evolution of viral escape mutations.

Conclusion

To conclude, several novel aspects about the role of virus-specific T cells emerged from recent studies in experimentally infected chimpanzees. In acute HBV infection, it has been clearly demonstrated that $CD8^+$ T cells are required for viral clearance and mediate disease pathogenesis. HBV-specific $CD8^+$ cells perform two antiviral functions that overlap temporally: an early primarily noncytolytic mechanism that may be mediated by IFN-γ and a primarily cytolytic mechanism that finally clears the remaining infected cells. In contrast, $CD4^+$ cells probably do not function as effector cells in the control of HBV since depletion of $CD4^+$ cells had little or no effect on the duration of the infection. However, since $CD4^+$ cells may play an early immunoregulatory role and since the depletion of $CD4^+$ cells was first performed in week 6, it is impossible to make a final statement about the role of $CD4^+$ cells in the outcome of HBV infection. Clearly, additional studies are required to define the role of $CD4^+$ T cells in HBV infection.

The intrahepatic virus-specific T-cell response is essential for the control of acute HCV infection since viral clearance or control is associated with the accumulation of HCV-specific $CD4^+$ and $CD8^+$ T cells in the liver. Importantly, viral clearance could occur in the absence of liver disease but in the presence of IFN-γ in the liver suggesting that IFN-γ might perform direct antiviral effector functions during acute HCV infection, similar to its ability to control HBV replication. This cytokine is probably secreted by virus-specific T cells that accumulate in the liver.

Combined virus-specific $CD4^+$ and $CD8^+$ T-cell responses are also required for the control of HCV rechallenge. Depletion studies could clearly demonstrate that $CD8^+$ T cells are the effector cells but that $CD4^+$ T cells are also necessary for the maintenance of a functional $CD8^+$ T-cell response. Studies in chimpanzees also revealed that different mechanisms contribute to the development of viral persistence such as the development of viral escape mutations and the failure of T cells to accumulate in the liver. However, much more work will be needed before the mechanisms responsible for viral clearance and persistence are fully understood. That knowledge is essential for the rational development of effective immunotherapy for chronic HCV infection.

Acknowledgments

The authors thank Keith Reiman and John Ghrayeb for providing monoclonal antihuman CD8 and CD4 antibodies, respectively, for the depletion experiments, and Carola Steiger and Max Shapiro for excellent technical assistance with the chimpanzee experiments. The work described in this review was supported by grants R01-CA76403 and R01-AI20001 from the National Institutes of Health (USA) and by a fellowship from the

Cancer Research Institute. R.T. is currently supported by grants from the Deutsche Forschungsgemeinschaft Th719 2-1 and 2-2 (Emmy Noether Programm), HepNet, and the Wilhelm Sander Foundation.

References

1 Rehermann B, Lau D, Hoofnagle JH, Chisari FV: Cytotoxic T lymphocyte responsiveness after resolution of chronic hepatitis B virus infection. J Clin Invest 1996;97:1655–1665.

2 Rehermann B, Fowler P, Sidney J, Person J, Redeker A, Brown M, Moss B, Sette A, Chisari FV: The cytotoxic T lymphocyte response to multiple hepatitis B virus polymerase epitopes during and after acute viral hepatitis. J Exp Med 1995;181:1047–1058.

3 Rehermann B, Ferrari C, Pasquinelli C, Chisari FV: The hepatitis B virus persists for decades after patients' recovery from acute viral hepatitis despite active maintenance of a cytotoxic T-lymphocyte response. Nat Med 1996;2:1104–1108.

4 Maini MK, Boni C, Ogg GS, King AS, Reignat S, Lee CK, Larrubia JR, Webster GJ, McMichael AJ, Ferrari C, Williams R, Vergani D, Bertoletti A: Direct ex vivo analysis of hepatitis B virus-specific CD8(+) T cells associated with the control of infection. Gastroenterology 1999;117:1386–1396.

5 Chisari FV: Cytotoxic T cells and viral hepatitis. J Clin Invest 1997;99:1472–1477.

6 Guidotti LG, Chisari FV: Noncytolytic control of viral infections by the innate and adaptive immune response. Annu Rev Immunol 2001;19:65–91.

7 Guidotti LG, Ishikawa T, Hobbs MV, Matzke B, Schreiber R, Chisari FV: Intracellular inactivation of the hepatitis B virus by cytotoxic T lymphocytes. Immunity 1996;4:25–36.

8 Barker LF, Maynard JE, Purcell RH, Hoofnagle JH, Berquist KR, London WT, Gerety RJ, Krushak DH: Hepatitis B virus infection in chimpanzees: Titration of subtypes. J Infect Dis 1975;132:451–458.

9 Guidotti LG, Rochford R, Chung J, Shapiro M, Purcell R, Chisari FV: Viral clearance without destruction of infected cells during acute HBV infection. Science 1999;284:825–829.

10 Bertoni R, Sette A, Sidney J, Guidotti LG, Shapiro M, Purcell R, Chisari FV: Human class I supertypes and CTL repertoires extend to chimpanzees. J Immunol 1998;161:4447–4455.

11 Thimme R, Wieland S, Steiger C, Ghrayeb J, Reimann KA, Purcell RH, Chisari FV: CD8(+) T cells mediate viral clearance and disease pathogenesis during acute hepatitis B virus infection. J Virol 2003;77:68–76.

12 Wieland S, Thimme R, Purcell RH, Chisari FV: Genomic analysis of the host response to hepatitis B virus infection. Proc Natl Acad Sci USA 2004;20:20.

13 Schmitz JE, Kuroda MJ, Santra S, Sasseville VG, Simon MA, Lifton MA, Racz P, Tenner-Racz K, Dalesandro M, Scallon BJ, Ghrayeb J, Forman MA, Montefiori DC, Rieber EP, Letvin NL, Reimann KA: Control of viremia in simian immunodeficiency virus infection by CD8+ lymphocytes. Science 1999;283:857–860.

14 Jonker M, Slingerland W, Treacy G, van Eerd P, Pak KY, Wilson E, Tam S, Bakker K, Lobuglio AF, Rieber P, et al: In vivo treatment with a monoclonal chimeric anti-CD4 antibody results in prolonged depletion of circulating CD4+ cells in chimpanzees. Clin Exp Immunol 1993;93: 301–307.

15 Diepolder HM, Zachoval R, Hoffmann RM, Wierenga EA, Santantonio T, Jung MC, Eichenlaub D, Pape GR: Possible mechanism involving T-lymphocyte response to non-structural protein 3 in viral clearance in acute hepatitis C virus infection. Lancet 1995;346:1006–1007.

16 Gerlach JT, Diepolder HM, Jung MC, Gruener NH, Schraut WW, Zachoval R, Hoffmann R, Schirren CA, Santantonio T, Pape GR: Recurrence of hepatitis C virus after loss of virus-specific CD4(+) T-cell response in acute hepatitis C. Gastroenterology 1999;117:933–941.

17 Gruner NH, Gerlach TJ, Jung MC, Diepolder HM, Schirren CA, Schraut WW, Hoffmann R, Zachoval R, Santantonio T, Cucchiarini M, Cerny A, Pape GR: Association of hepatitis C virus-specific CD8+ T cells with viral clearance in acute hepatitis C. J Infect Dis 2000;181:1528–1536.

18 Lechner F, Wong DK, Dunbar PR, Chapman R, Chung RT, Dohrenwend P, Robbins G, Phillips R, Klenerman P, Walker BD: Analysis of successful immune responses in persons infected with hepatitis C virus. J Exp Med 2000;191:1499–1512.
19 Thimme R, Oldach D, Chang KM, Steiger C, Ray SC, Chisari FV: Determinants of viral clearance and persistence during acute hepatitis C virus infection. J Exp Med 2001;194:1395–1406.
20 Bukh J, Forns X, Emerson SU, Purcell RH: Studies of hepatitis C virus in chimpanzees and their importance for vaccine development. Intervirology 2001;44:132–142.
21 Cooper S, Erickson AL, Adams EJ, Kansopon J, Weiner AJ, Chien DY, Houghton M, Parham P, Walker CM: Analysis of a successful immune response against hepatitis C virus. Immunity 1999;10:439–449.
22 Frese M, Schwarzle V, Barth K, Krieger N, Lohmann V, Mihm S, Haller O, Bartenschlager R: Interferon-γ inhibits replication of subgenomic and genomic hepatitis C virus RNAs. Hepatology 2002;35:694–703.
23 Liu C, Zhu H, Tu Z, Xu YL, Nelson DR: CD8+ T-cell interaction with HCV replicon cells: Evidence for both cytokine- and cell-mediated antiviral activity. Hepatology 2003;37:1335–1342.
24 Su AI, Pezacki JP, Wodicka L, Brideau AD, Supekova L, Thimme R, Wieland S, Bukh J, Purcell RH, Schultz PG, Chisari FV: Genomic analysis of the host response to hepatitis C virus infection. Proc Natl Acad Sci USA 2002;99:15669–15674.
25 Thomson M, Nascimbeni M, Havert MB, Major M, Gonzales S, Alter H, Feinstone SM, Murthy KK, Rehermann B, Liang TJ: The clearance of hepatitis C virus infection in chimpanzees may not necessarily correlate with the appearance of acquired immunity. J Virol 2003;77:862–870.
26 Erickson AL, Kimura Y, Igarashi S, Eichelberger J, Houghton M, Sidney J, McKinney D, Sette A, Hughes AL, Walker C: The outcome of hepatitis C virus infection is predicted by escape mutations in epitopes targeted by cytotoxic T lymphocytes. Immunity 2001;15:885–895.
27 Thimme R, Bukh J, Spangenberg HC, Wieland S, Pemberton J, Steiger C, Govindarajan S, Purcell RH, Chisari FV: Viral and immunological determinants of hepatitis C virus clearance, persistence, and disease. Proc Natl Acad Sci USA 2002;99:15661–15668.
28 Prince AM, Brotman B, Huima T, Pascual D, Jaffery M, Inchauspe G: Immunity in hepatitis C infection. J Infect Dis 1992;165:438–443.
29 Farci P, Alter HJ, Govindarajan S, Wong DC, Engle R, Lesniewski RR, Mushahwar IK, Desai SM, Miller RH, Ogata N, et al: Lack of protective immunity against reinfection with hepatitis C virus. Science 1992;258:135–140.
30 Bassett SE, Guerra B, Brasky K, Miskovsky E, Houghton M, Klimpel GR, Lanford RE: Protective immune response to hepatitis C virus in chimpanzees rechallenged following clearance of primary infection. Hepatology 2001;33:1479–1487.
31 Major ME, Mihalik K, Puig M, Rehermann B, Nascimbeni M, Rice CM, Feinstone SM: Previously infected and recovered chimpanzees exhibit rapid responses that control hepatitis C virus replication upon rechallenge. J Virol 2002;76:6586–6595.
32 Weiner AJ, Paliard X, Selby MJ, Medina-Selby A, Coit D, Nguyen S, Kansopon J, Arian CL, Ng P, Tucker J, Lee CT, Polakos NK, Han J, Wong S, Lu HH, Rosenberg S, Brasky KM, Chien D, Kuo G, Houghton M: Intrahepatic genetic inoculation of hepatitis C virus RNA confers cross-protective immunity. J Virol 2001;75:7142–7148.
33 Shoukry NH, Grakoui A, Houghton M, Chien DY, Ghrayeb J, Reimann KA, Walker CM: Memory CD8+ T cells are required for protection from persistent hepatitis C virus infection. J Exp Med 2003;197:1645–1655.
34 Grakoui A, Shoukry NH, Woollard DJ, Han JH, Hanson HL, Ghrayeb J, Murthy KK, Rice CM, Walker CM: HCV persistence and immune evasion in the absence of memory T cell help. Science 2003;302:659–662.

R. Thimme
Department of Medicine II, University of Freiburg
Hugstetterstrasse 55, DE–79106 Freiburg (Germany)
Tel. +49 761 2703758, Fax +49 761 2703372, E-Mail thimme@med1.ukl.uni-freiburg.de

von Weizsäcker F, Roggendorf M (eds): Models of Viral Hepatitis.
Monogr Virol. Basel, Karger, 2005, vol 25, pp 81–95

The Replicon System as an Efficient Tool to Study HCV RNA Replication

Volker Lohmann

Department of Molecular Virology, University of Heidelberg,
Heidelberg, Germany

Hepatitis C virus (HCV) is an enveloped virus with a plus-strand RNA genome of ca. 9.6 kb in length. It is classified into the genus Hepacivirus of the *Flaviviridae* [1] and, due to its high genetic diversity, further divided into six genotypes (1–6) each consisting of several subtypes (a, b, etc.) [2]. The genome contains one long open reading frame, encoding a polyprotein of approximately 3,000 amino acids length, which is flanked by nontranslated regions (NTRs, fig. 1a). The 5′ NTR mediates translation of the polyprotein by an internal ribosome entry site (IRES) [3] and has as well as the 3′ NTR an important role for viral RNA replication [4–8]. The polyprotein is co- and post-translationally cleaved by viral and host-cell proteases into its functional subunits core (C), envelope protein 1 (E1), E2, p7, nonstructural protein 2 (NS2), NS3, NS4A, NS4B, NS5A and NS5B [reviewed in 9]. Core, E1 and E2 are the major constituents of the virus particle. Recent data imply that p7 might act as a viroporin [10, 11]. NS3 is the key viral protease that in conjunction with NS2 is required for NS2–3 cleavage, and, after association with its cofactor NS4A, processes all downstream cleavage sites. In addition, the C-terminal part of NS3 harbors a helicase activity. Replication takes place in a specialized membrane compartment called the 'membranous web' which is induced by NS4B [12, 13]. NS5A is a highly phosphorylated protein that has been implicated in the resistance of HCV to interferon-α [reviewed in 14] and that is involved in cell culture adaptation [15, 16]. Finally, NS5B is the RNA-dependent RNA polymerase (RdRp), the catalytic core of the HCV replication complex.

In 1989 the HCV genome was first cloned and identified as the major cause of nonA-nonB hepatitis [17]. Numerous groups have tried to establish

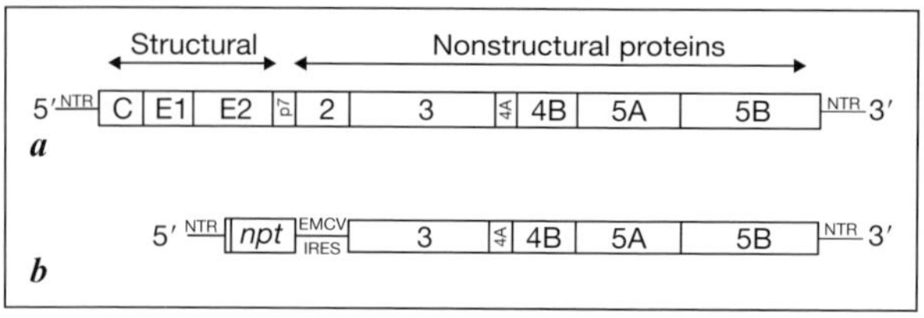

Fig. 1. Schematic representation of the HCV genome (***a***) and the structure of subgenomic replicons (***b***). *npt*, gene encoding neomycin phosphotransferase, EMCV IRES, internal ribosome entry site of the encephalomyocarditis virus.

cell culture systems for HCV, but up to now there is still no efficient way to propagate the virus ex vivo. All cell culture systems described thus far, including primary hepatocytes, rely on highly sensitive methods for the detection of HCV replication [reviewed in 18]. The situation has changed during the last years by the development of subgenomic HCV replicons [19]. The aim of this chapter is to give an overview of the principles and applications of the HCV replicon system.

Principles of the Replicon System and Properties of Selected Cell Clones

For many plus-strand RNA viruses it has been shown that in vitro transcribed RNA encompassing the complete genome is infectious and directs the production of virus particles after transfection into permissive host cells [20]. Such a system has several advantages compared to the infection of cells with patient sera: (i) no cellular receptor is required, which often limits the delivery of the genome into a cell; (ii) cloned viral genomes are well defined and can be produced from cloned cDNA in huge amounts by in vitro transcription; (iii) once such a system works, it allows the systematic analysis of the effect of mutations in the viral genome. For many viruses this approach was straightforward, but in the case of HCV a major problem was the lack of a cell culture system to monitor replication. Therefore, it took 8 years after the first cloning of HCV to generate transcripts from cloned cDNA that were shown to be infectious by intrahepatic inoculation in chimpanzees [21, 22]. The success was based on the construction of isolate-specific consensus genomes, thereby minimizing the probability of deleterious mutations in individually cloned variants. Unfortunately, after this important breakthrough it turned out that these infectious cloned HCV genomes seemed not to replicate after transfection into cultured cells. However, given the low efficiency of HCV replication in infected cells and the huge amount of input RNA in a transfection experiment, it would technically be almost impossible to detect low level viral replication in this experimental setting. To overcome these problems, we constructed subgenomic replicons based on a patient-derived consensus isolate, designated Con1, which was cloned in our laboratory [19, 23]. The principal concept was to replace the sequence of the structural proteins by a selectable marker gene (*npt*, encoding neomycin phosphotransferase) and to insert a second IRES element to allow translation of the nonstructural proteins NS3 to NS5B (fig. 1b), which have been shown in other virus systems to be necessary and sufficient for replication [24, 25]. Upon transfection of these subgenomic, selectable replicons into permissive host cells and selection with G418, only those cells would survive and divide which produced npt in sufficient amounts by multiplication of the replicons to withstand the selective pressure. In case of Huh-7, a human hepatoma cell line, we were able to obtain a low number of cell colonies by this approach that could be expanded to cell clones [19]. The most striking feature of these clones was an unexpectedly high level of replication with about 1,000 replicon copies per cell, allowing the application of standard methods like Northern and Western blot for the detection of viral RNA and antigens. Immunofluorescence studies revealed that almost all cells in replicon cell clones expressed detectable amounts of the HCV NS proteins in the cytoplasm in a punctuated, ER-like staining pattern. In principle, replicon cell clones can be passaged indefinitely with growth rates not distinguishable from naive Huh-7 cells. Furthermore, replicon cells show no obvious morphological changes or signs of cytopathogenicity, indicating that persistent HCV replication is tolerated well by the host cell. However, detailed ultrastructural analyses identified morphological modifications of the ER, resembling alterations observed in liver biopsies of HCV-infected individuals [26] and specific membrane structures, designated the membranous web, that have been shown to be the site of RNA replication [13].

Determinants of Replication Efficiency of the Con1 Isolate

In contrast to the high HCV replication rate in selected replicon cell clones, the efficiency with which these clones were established was originally extremely low. Transfection of 1 μg replicon RNA, representing ca. 2×10^{11} molecules, into 4 million Huh-7 cells yielded at best 20–40 G418-resistant replicon cell clones. Meanwhile it has been shown that two major determinants account for this striking discrepancy: (i) The Con1 wild-type isolate replicates poorly in Huh-7 cells and has to acquire adaptive mutations that enhance replication efficiency to a level that is sufficient to confer resistance to G418 selection. (ii) Only a minor subpopulation of the Huh-7 cells supports the persistent

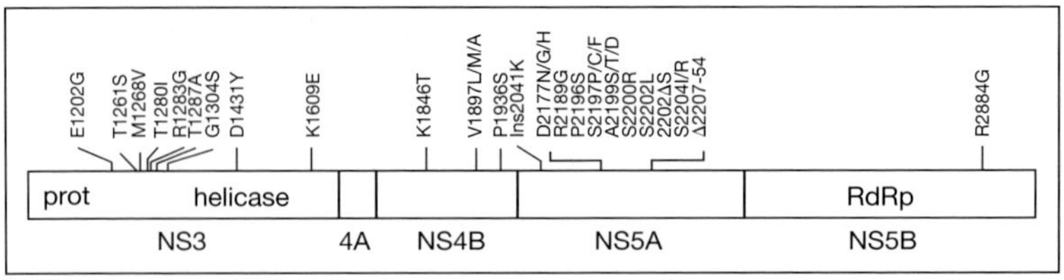

Fig. 2. Location of adaptive mutations identified in replicon cell clones derived from the HCV Con1 genome [15, 16, 27–29, 54]. Numbers refer to the amino acid positions of the Con1 polyprotein.

high level HCV replication which is robust enough to permit cell growth under the applied selective pressure. Both mechanisms will be described in more detail in the following paragraphs.

First it was shown by several groups that the sequence of the HCV nonstructural proteins in selected replicon cell clones had acquired conserved mutations not present in the replicons that were introduced into the cells. When these mutations were transferred back into the original Con1 replicon sequence, the efficiency of colony formation increased significantly [15, 16, 27, 28]. Such adaptive mutations were identified in almost all nonstructural proteins of the Con1 isolate, with particular clusterings at the N-terminus of the NS3 helicase, at two positions within NS4B (K1846 and V1897) and especially in the center of NS5A, encompassing amino acids 2177–2204 (fig. 2). This region has been shown to be important for hyperphosphorylation of NS5A, but up to now it was not possible to demonstrate a clear correlation between the phosphorylation state of NS5A and adaptation [15, 16]. Based on their impact on HCV replication and on cooperative effects, adaptive mutations can be classified into two groups: mutations in NS4B, NS5A and one particular substitution in NS5B enhance HCV replication significantly but lead to a reduced replication rate when combined with one another in cis [29]. The second group includes mutations in NS3 that have a minor effect on HCV replication when analyzed individually, but cooperatively increase replication when combined with adaptive mutations from the first group [29]. The most efficient Con1 variant generated so far in our laboratory therefore contains two mutations in NS3 (E1202G and T1280I) and one mutation in NS4B (K1846T). The molecular basics underlying adaptation of the Con1 genome to Huh-7 cells remain to be determined but it seems plausible that the interaction with particular host factors might be modulated by adaptive mutations.

The second major determinant for efficient HCV replication in Huh-7 is the host cell itself. Transient HCV replication assays revealed more than 100-fold differences in permissiveness between different passages of naive Huh-7 cells even when they are generated from the same stock [29]. In addition, after the removal of replicons from selected cell clones by treatment with IFNs or selective drugs, some of the 'cured' Huh-7 clones are more permissive for HCV replication compared to naive cells [30, 31]. Therefore, establishment of replicon cell clones includes selection not only for adaptive mutations but also for permissive host cells. The permissiveness of the cell can even compensate for the effect of viral adaptation, since several Con1 replicon clones have been described showing no adaptive mutations in the HCV sequence [15]. One of these clones showed a significantly increased permissiveness after removal of the replicon compared to naive Huh-7 cells [30].

It is very difficult to compare the permissiveness of naive Huh-7 cells and cured replicon clones used in different laboratories, since the data rely on various assays. However, it is well established that the host cells, as well as the usage of appropriate adaptive mutations, are both critical determinants for the establishment of replicon cell clones and transient replication assays [15, 29–32]. In contrast, once a replicon cell clone is established, the level of persistent replication is rather similar between different cell clones, replicons carrying various adaptive mutations and in different laboratories and seems to be regulated by a complex interplay between the host cell and the replicon, which is dictated by the applied selective pressure.

HCV Isolates Successfully Used in the Replicon System

The infectious Con1 genome is an isolate-specific consensus sequence cloned from the total liver RNA of an infected patient and is classified into genotype 1b. Up to now, four other genotype 1b isolates (HCV-N [27, 33], HCV-BK [34], 1B-1 [35] 1B-2R1[32]) and one isolate of genotype 1a [34, 36, 37] were successfully used to generate subgenomic replicons. HCV-N is a cloned patient isolate previously shown to be infectious by intrahepatic inoculation of chimpanzees with low efficiency [38]. Interestingly, the initial replication capacity of replicons derived from this sequence was high compared to nonadapted Con1 replicons [27, 33]. A unique four amino acid insertion in NS5A (SSYN at position 2219), close to site where many adaptive mutations in Con1 are located (fig. 2), was shown to be required for this phenotype. Therefore, the insertion found in HCV-N confers cell culture adaptation and in turn may lead to attenuation in chimpanzees. A similar inverse correlation between replication capacity in vivo and in vitro was observed with the Con1 isolate [39]. The Con1 wild-type isolate replicated well after intrahepatic inoculation of chimpanzees, whereas a highly adapted variant containing three mutations (E1202G, T1280I, S2197P) was unable to establish a productive infection. If only one mutation was included (S2197P), the genome retained its infectivity, but the whole virus population in the blood was reverted to the wild-type sequence, arguing for an inverse correlation between replication in Huh-7 cells and in vivo [39].

Replicons from all other isolates successfully tested so far either had acquired adaptive mutations after selection of replicon cell clones [32, 35], or could only be established by the introduction of such an adaptive mutation into the replicon sequence [34, 36, 37].

In case of HCV 1B-1, an HCV genotype 1b consensus isolate was generated from MT-2 cells infected with an HCV-positive patient serum and used for the construction of selectable replicons. Only one Huh-7 cell clone was established with this isolate having adaptive mutations in NS3 and NS4B (K1609E, V1896P [35]).

Another functional genotype 1b replicon was obtained from infected PH5CH8 cells by cloning a whole NS3 to NS5B-variant library into a replicon cassette vector to keep the quasispecies diversity [32]. A single replicon cell clone was obtained with this strategy, designated 1B-2R1, again having acquired particular mutations in NS3 and NS5A (I1380F and S2200R). Although not very efficient in this case, the generation of quasispecies libraries might be an alternative to obtain functional HCV isolates replicating in cell culture that is less difficult and time consuming than the construction of consensus genomes. In addition, having a consensus genome is no guarantee for successful replication in cell culture, as exemplified by the genotype 1a H77 isolate, which is infectious in chimpanzees [21]. Several groups have tried to generate subgenomic replicons from this isolate without success [15, 27]. Only after introduction of an adaptive mutation (S2204I) and by using highly permissive Huh-7 cells was it possible to generate a few cell clones harboring replicons derived from this genome. All analyzed cell clones had an additional mutation within NS3, either A1226D or P1496L, which was required for efficient replication. Interestingly, amino acid 1496 was also a key determinant for HCV-BK replicons, an infectious genotype 1b genome [34]. Even after introduction of the S2204I mutation, replicons based on this isolate were not functional. Chimeras with the Con1 nonstructural protein sequences revealed the critical determinant within NS3. After individually exchanging every amino acid in NS3 deviating from Con1, it was shown that S1222 and R1496 in the BK sequence independently blocked replication and that conversion of either one of these sites to the Con1 sequence (S1222T or R1496M) restored replication of HCV-BK-derived replicons [34]. Position 1496 is particularly interesting since considerable heterogeneity exists at this site in published HCV sequences, with about 25% having an arginine, which is at least for HCV-BK deleterious for replication and also impairs replication of Con1 in cell culture [34]. However, for the H77 isolate a cell line could be generated with a chimeric replicon, harboring the N-terminal 75 amino acids of NS3 from Con1 combined with the NS-protein sequence of H77, with no changes at position 1496 but with the mutations S1358P and K1609E [37], emphasizing the important and complex role of NS3 for efficient HCV replication in cell culture.

Although currently six independent isolates of HCV genotype 1 efficiently replicate in the replicon system, it is still hard to predict if a given genome is capable of efficient replication in Huh-7 cells and what the requirements for the generation of replicons from other genotypes are. At least for genotype 1, the mechanism underlying adaptation seems to be conserved, since those mutations tested so far enhance replication of all isolates (e.g. S2204I for Con1, H77, HCV-N and BK [15, 33, 34]). Therefore, the same mutations can most likely be used to enhance replication of other genotype 1 isolates. In addition, some positions in NS3 (e.g. 1496) seem to be very critical [34, 36]. The situation is further complicated by the apparent negative correlation between replication in cell culture and in the chimpanzee system, which is apart from replicons currently the only efficient functional assay for the replication capacity of a cloned HCV isolate.

Cell Lines Permissive for HCV Replicons

A very critical question refers to the host cell requirements for efficient HCV replication in cell culture. For several years, Huh-7 was the only cell line supporting HCV replication in the replicon system and many attempts failed to establish persistent replicons in other cell types. The narrow host range and the tropism of HCV, which indicated the requirement for a particular host cell environment, were believed to be responsible for the restriction to Huh-7 cells. This view was challenged by the development of replicon cell clones derived from HeLa and Hepa1–6 cells, a mouse hepatoma cell line [40]. Interestingly, the authors failed in both cases to obtain cell clones by transfection of in vitro transcribed replicons with a defined sequence. It was only when total cellular RNA from a Huh-7 replicon cell clone was transfected that colonies arose after G418 selection in case of HeLa cells. In case of the mouse hepatoma cells, colony formation was restricted to the use of total RNA from the newly established HeLa replicon clones, arguing for specific mutations required for efficient replication in HeLa and Hepa1–6 cells, which are present in the replicon quasispecies by chance. Sequence analysis of the replicons in HeLa and mouse hepatoma cells revealed several mutations, especially in NS5A and NS4B, with one particular NS4B variation, V1749A, being conserved in all analyzed HeLa and mouse hepatoma replicon clones. However, by introduction of this and other mutations into cloned replicons it was up to now not possible to define the sequence determinants for adaptation to HeLa and mouse hepatoma cells.

In addition to necessary adaptive mutations, only a minor subpopulation of the cells might be permissive for HCV replication, as was shown for Huh-7 [29–31], and thereby limit the efficiency of colony formation.

The major lesson from the established Hepa1–6 and HeLa replicon cells is that replication of HCV in the replicon system does not seem to be limited by liver-specific host factors but by a yet undefined mechanism that remains to be elucidated. On the other hand, narrow host range and tropism in vivo might be determined primarily by virus entry and assembly and not by factors required for replication. Interestingly, none of the cell lines reported to support HCV replication after inoculation with patient sera [reviewed in 18], like MT-2 or PH5CH8, have been shown to work in the replicon system. Since the establishment of replicon cells requires a certain amount of npt to confer resistance to G418, most cell lines not permissive for replicons might not allow or tolerate the sufficiently high HCV replication level.

Applications of Replicon Cell Clones and Transient Replication Assays

Many different questions related to the life cycle of HCV can be addressed by the replicon system and in principal two tools exist that differ in their applicability depending on the experimental needs: selected replicon cell clones and transient replication assays.

Selected replicon cell clones show high level, persistent HCV replication in almost all cells of a given population, which is kept by constant selection with G418. Replication can be monitored by many robust assays, like Northern blot or quantitative RT-PCR for RNA detection and Western blot or immunofluorescence for antigen detection [15, 19, 41]. More recent advances include cell clones containing a replicon expressing a firefly luciferase/ubiquitin/npt fusion protein instead of npt, that allow the quantitation of HCV replication by simple luciferase assays in cell lysates [42, 43] or replicon cell clones inducing the expression of secreted alkaline phophatase as a measure of HCV replication [44]. For some experiments the bicistronic nature of the 'classical' replicons could be a problem (fig. 1b), because the translation of the HCV NS proteins by the EMCV-IRES might have an impact on the results, e.g. in studies on the mechanism of IFN. Therefore, cell lines carrying monocistronic replicons were generated, in which the selection marker is fused by ubiquitin to the N-terminus of NS3 [42]. Furthermore, cell clones have been established expressing the whole HCV polyprotein [30, 33, 45]. Although these cells should principally be able to produce virus particles, for unknown reasons up to now no significant secretion of virions was observed.

Replicon cell clones are the optimal tool whenever a constantly high level of replication is required without the need to manipulate the HCV sequence. Therefore the major topics analyzed with selected replicon cell clones are screening and evaluation of antiviral drugs [e.g. 46–49], the effect of IFN on HCV replication [e.g. 27, 50–55], biochemical analyses on the viral replicase complex [e.g. 56–60], ultrastructural analyses [e.g. 13, 26] and virus host cell interactions [e.g. 61–66]. Selected replicon cell clones are available for all cell types and isolates described above.

However, selected replicon cell clones are not applicable to reverse genetic studies because this requires the possibility to alter the HCV sequence, which is not possible after establishment of a cell clone. Hence, transient replication assays have been established, allowing the quantitation of the replication efficiency of given replicon RNAs. The critical determinants for all transient replication assays are the type of adaptive mutations, the permissiveness of the Huh-7 cells and the method used to quantify replication [15, 16, 29–31]. The simplest 'transient' replication assay uses selectable replicons (fig. 1b) and quantifies the efficiency of colony formation after transfection and selection by counting the number of selected colonies per microgram of transfected RNA or relative to the amount of transfected cells [e.g. 15, 28]. This kind of assay has the advantage of being relatively sensitive and robust. The main disadvantages are the time required for selection of colonies, typically 3–4 weeks, and the quantitation by manual counting, which is very time consuming and error prone, since not every colony represents a viable cell clone.

Another type of transient replication assay is based on the detection of HCV RNA early after transfection either by quantitative RT-PCR [e.g. 15, 30] or Northern blot [e.g., 16, 45], thereby eliminating the need for any foreign sequences like selectable markers or reporter genes and allowing even analyses of in vitro transcribed full-length genomes [30, 36, 39, 45]. The drawback of Northern blot assays is a limited sensitivity, which restricts the analysis to highly cell culture-adapted HCV sequences. In case of RT-PCR assays, the plasmid DNA used to generate the replicons has to be rigorously removed prior to transfection, because it would produce a long-lasting background due to the higher stability of DNA compared to RNA and the lack of discrimination between DNA and RNA by the assay.

The easiest and fastest approach to measure HCV replication early after transfection is based on replicons with reporter genes instead of selectable markers. The first reporter replicons contained the firefly luciferase, which provides a very low cellular background, a high sensitivity and a short half-life; therefore, luciferase activity in cell lysates reflects RNA replication well [16]. The system was further optimized by including a poliovirus IRES element to initiate translation of the reporter gene instead of the HCV IRES [5, 29]. Another reporter system relies on the expression of an HIV-tat/picornavirus 2A proteinase/npt fusion protein in a replicon transfected into Huh-7 cells stably harboring the gene for secreted alkaline phosphatase (SEAP) under translational control of the HIV-LTR promoter [44]. Therefore, tat is produced upon HCV replication, leading to the production of SEAP, which can be quantified in the supernatant of the cells as a correlate of HCV replication. The system has the advantage to monitor HCV replication in the cell culture supernatant, but since SEAP is expressed via activation of a nuclear promoter by HIV-tat, the analysis is rather indirect and might be prone to artifacts. The most recently published reporter replicon uses the bacterial β-lactamase gene (bla) [31], offering the opportunity to stain living cells with a substrate that is metabolized by the reporter protein, thereby changing its fluorescent color from green to blue. Hence, replication can be quantified as percent blue cells or by measuring total bla activity in a cell lysate.

Transient HCV replication assays have been involved in several studies, including the analysis of adaptive mutations [e.g. 15, 16, 27–29, 54], the characterization of different HCV isolates [e.g. 33, 34, 36], the role of the HCV NTRs [5–8, 67], the structure function analysis of HCV NS5B [68, 69] and NS5A [70, 71] and the permissiveness of Huh-7 cells [29–31]. In contrast to replicon cell clones, which are extremely robust with high levels of persistent replication, transient assays are in general technically more difficult and less reproducible, since the total readout depends on many determinants, among which transfection efficiency, HCV isolate and adaptive mutations used, permissiveness of the Huh-7 cells and type of transient assay are the most important. As a general guideline, colony formation assays are most sensitive and robust, but time consuming and hard to quantify, especially with poorly replicating replicons. Reporter assays are fastest and easiest to perform and to quantify, but require a careful setup to show that reporter activity indeed correlates with RNA replication. RNA detection assays give a direct measurement of RNA replication, providing the only option when additional marker genes are not desired, but are technically difficult and require most hand on time per assay. Transient replication assays are currently restricted to Huh-7 cells and cannot be used for HeLa or mouse hepatoma cells. It is hard to judge which isolate is most efficient in transient assays, since no careful side-by-side analysis with the most efficient replicons established in different laboratories has been performed. Most studies published up to now use Con1 with different combinations of adaptive mutations [e.g. 15, 16, 29].

Perspectives and Limitations

HCV replicons are still the only efficient cell culture system allowing the study of HCV replication with robust and reliable biochemical means of antigen and RNA detection. They allow for the first time extensive genetic studies on HCV and have already been exploited for detailed analyses on the role of the NTRs in RNA replication and to characterize the role of adaptive mutations. Replicon cell clones provide an excellent tool for the screening and evaluation of specific antiviral drugs and allow the detailed biochemical and ultrastructural analysis of the HCV replication complex and the cellular requirements for HCV replication. Several potential cellular factors have already been identified in yeast two-hybrid screens and can now be evaluated for their biological significance (e.g. VAP-A [72]). However, to exclude clonal variations, all experiments dealing with host cell interactions should be done with several independent replicon cell clones. In addition, HeLa and Hepa1–6 replicon cell lines are now available for comparative analyses to exclude possible cell type-specific artifacts of Huh-7 cells [40].

The major limitation of the replicon system is the lack of virion production. No secretion of virus particles has been observed yet, either with selectable replicon clones harboring the complete HCV ORF, or after transient transfection of vitro transcribed full-length genomes [33, 45]. It is still obscure if this is due to restrictions of the host cells or due to assembly incompetence of the structural proteins. The latter would indicate that assembly might be impaired by cell culture adaptation, since all isolates tested for particle production in the replicon system are infectious in chimpanzees, as a proof of assembly competence in vivo. In this scenario it would be hard to get efficient replication in a cell culture system that is fully permissive for the whole HCV life cycle. If Huh-7 cells are limiting particle production, the newly established HeLa- and Hepa1–6 cells might provide a solution for this problem. Until this road block is removed, studies on aspects of HCV multiplication aside from RNA replication are restricted to infectable cell lines or primary cells, like tupaia primary hepatocytes, which are also described in this book. In addition, retroviruses pseudotyped with the HCV glycoproteins E1 and E2 have recently been established allowing the analysis of some aspects of virus attachment and entry [73].

In summary, the study of the HCV life cycle in cell culture still is a challenging task, but replicons currently provide the most efficient tool to analyze almost all aspects on RNA replication in a cellular environment.

Acknowledgement

Thanks to Ralf Bartenschlager for critically editing the manuscript.

References

1 Van Regenmortel MHV, Fauquet CM, Bishop DHL, Carstens EB, Estes MK, Lemon SM, Maniloff J, Mayo MA, McGeoch DJ, Pringle CR, Wickner RB: Virus taxonomy: The VIIth Report of the International Committee on Taxonomy of Viruses. San Diego, Academic Press, 2000.
2 Simmonds P, Holmes EC, Cha TA, Chan SW, McOmish F, Irvine B, Beall E, Yap PL, Kolberg J, Urdea MS: Classification of hepatitis C virus into six major genotypes and a series of subtypes by phylogenetic analysis of the NS-5 region. J Gen Virol 1993;74:2391–2399.
3 Tsukiyama KK, Iizuka N, Kohara M, Nomoto A: Internal ribosome entry site within hepatitis C virus RNA. J Virol 1992;66:1476–1483.
4 Kolykhalov AA, Mihalik K, Feinstone SM, Rice CM: Hepatitis C virus-encoded enzymatic activities and conserved RNA elements in the 3′ nontranslated region are essential for virus replication in vivo. J Virol 2000;74:2046–2051.
5 Friebe P, Lohmann V, Krieger N, Bartenschlager R: Sequences in the 5′ nontranslated region of hepatitis C virus required for RNA replication. J Virol 2001;75:12047–12057.
6 Friebe P, Bartenschlager R: Genetic analysis of sequences in the 3′ nontranslated region of hepatitis C virus that are important for RNA replication. J Virol 2002;76:5326–5338.
7 Yi M, Lemon SM: Structure-function analysis of the 3′ stem-loop of hepatitis C virus genomic RNA and its role in viral RNA replication. RNA 2003;9:331–345.
8 Yi M, Lemon SM: 3′ nontranslated RNA signals required for replication of hepatitis C virus RNA. J Virol 2003;77:3557–3568.
9 Reed KE, Rice CM: Overview of hepatitis C virus genome structure, polyprotein processing, and protein properties. Curr Top Microbiol Immunol 2000;242:55–84.
10 Griffin SD, Beales LP, Clarke DS, Worsfold O, Evans SD, Jaeger J, Harris MP, Rowlands DJ: The p7 protein of hepatitis C virus forms an ion channel that is blocked by the antiviral drug, amantadine. FEBS Lett 2003;535:34–38.
11 Pavlovic D, Neville DC, Argaud O, Blumberg B, Dwek RA, Fischer WB, Zitzmann N: The hepatitis C virus p7 protein forms an ion channel that is inhibited by long-alkyl-chain iminosugar derivatives. Proc Natl Acad Sci USA 2003;100:6104–6108.
12 Egger D, Wolk B, Gosert R, Bianchi L, Blum HE, Moradpour D, Bienz K: Expression of hepatitis C virus proteins induces distinct membrane alterations including a candidate viral replication complex. J Virol 2002;76:5974–5984.
13 Gosert R, Egger D, Lohmann V, Bartenschlager R, Blum HE, Bienz K, Moradpour D: Identification of the hepatitis C virus RNA replication complex in Huh-7 cells harboring subgenomic replicons. J Virol 2003;77:5487–5492.
14 Khabar KS, Polyak SJ: Hepatitis C virus-host interactions: The NS5A protein and the interferon/chemokine systems. J Interferon Cytokine Res 2002;22:1005–1012.
15 Blight KJ, Kolykhalov AA, Rice CM: Efficient initiation of HCV RNA replication in cell culture. Science 2000;290:1972–1974.
16 Krieger N, Lohmann V, Bartenschlager R: Enhancement of hepatitis C virus RNA replication by cell culture-adaptive mutations. J Virol 2001;75:4614–4624.
17 Choo QL, Kuo G, Weiner AJ, Overby LR, Bradley DW, Houghton M: Isolation of a cDNA clone derived from a blood-borne non-A, non-B viral hepatitis genome. Science 1989;244:359–362.
18 Bartenschlager R, Lohmann V: Novel cell culture systems for the hepatitis C virus. Antiviral Res 2001;52:1–17.
19 Lohmann V, Körner F, Koch JO, Herian U, Theilmann L, Bartenschlager R: Replication of subgenomic hepatitis C virus RNAs in a hepatoma cell line. Science 1999;285:110–113.
20 Boyer JC, Haenni AL: Infectious transcripts and cDNA clones of RNA viruses. Virology 1994;198:415–426.
21 Kolykhalov AA, Agapov EV, Blight KJ, Mihalik K, Feinstone SM, Rice CM: Transmission of hepatitis C by intrahepatic inoculation with transcribed RNA. Science 1997;277:570–574.
22 Yanagi M, Purcell RH, Emerson SU, Bukh J: Transcripts from a single full-length cDNA clone of hepatitis C virus are infectious when directly transfected into the liver of a chimpanzee. Proc Natl Acad Sci USA 1997;94:8738–8743.

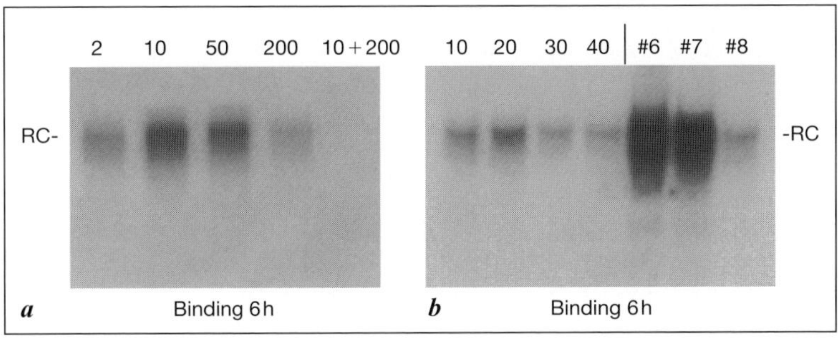

Fig. 1. ***a*** Binding of HBV to primary tupaia hepatocytes. The cells were seeded at confluence on a six-well culture dish as recently described [25]. HBV-positive human serum (2, 10, 50 and 200 μl) or a mixture of 10 μl HBV-positive serum with 200 μl of HBV-negative serum was added to the culture medium (1 ml/well). Viral titer in the HBV-positive serum was approximately 10^9 genomes/ml. The cells were incubated for 6 h at 37°C and subsequently washed extensively with culture medium. The cells were lysed in the culture dish; DNA was extracted and finally analyzed by Southern blotting. RC = Relaxed circular DNA originating from adherent HBV particles. ***b*** Effect of virus purification on viral attachment. HBV-positive serum (200 μl) was loaded on a gradient consisting of 10–60% Nycodenz dissolved in culture medium. Centrifugation was for 45 min with 55,000 rpm at 20°C in a TLS55 swing-out rotor. Virus containing fractions #6, #7 and #8 (150 μl each) were added to the culture medium covering the hepatocytes (right panel). Non-processed HBV-positive serum (10, 20, 30 and 40 μl) was added for reference (left panel). The cells were incubated for 6 h, washed and analyzed for viral DNA by Southern blotting.

To remove the inhibitory component, we processed the HBV-positive serum by gradient centrifugation. The iodinated benzoic acid derivative Nycodenz was chosen as a gradient medium because it is not toxic to tissue culture cells and it was used in former studies for the purification of active Epstein-Barr virus [9]. HBV particles prepared by gradient sedimentation efficiently bind to primary tupaia hepatocytes and the amount of cell-associated virus is strongly enhanced relative to the samples where HBV-positive serum was added directly to the culture dish (fig. 1b).

Purified HBV particles infect the primary hepatocytes as evidenced by the formation of covalently closed circular DNA (cccDNA) after 1 week in culture, whereas the cccDNA signal is hardly detectable for the cells infected with non-processed serum (fig. 2a). Inoculation of primary rat hepatocytes with purified viral particles does not result in cccDNA formation (fig. 2b). However, relaxed circular DNA (rcDNA) is detectable even after prolonged culture time. In addition, gradient-purified woodchuck hepatitis virus (WHV) binds to the cells but fails to infect primary hepatocytes from *T. belangeri*. Therefore, the hepadnaviral species tropism remains preserved after purification.

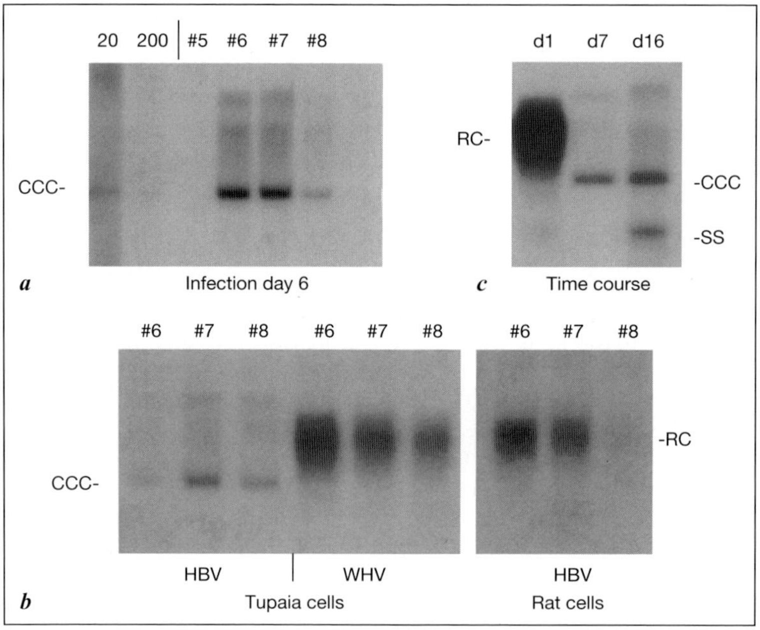

Fig. 2. ***a*** Infection with purified virions. Viral particles from 200 µl HBV-positive serum were purified by gradient sedimentation. Fractions #5, #6, #7 and #8 were applied to infect primary tupaia hepatocytes (right panel). Two wells were inoculated with 20 or 200 µl of non-processed HBV-positive serum (left panel). The cells were kept for 6 days at 37°C with culture medium being refreshed daily. Viral DNA was extracted from the cell lysate and visualized by Southern blotting. CCC = Covalently closed circular DNA. ***b*** Species tropism of viral infection. Primary hepatocytes were inoculated with gradient-purified HBV from human serum (left panel) or WHV from woodchuck serum (middle panel). Primary hepatocytes from rat were inoculated with purified HBV particles (right panel). The cells were harvested on day 6 post-infection and analyzed for viral DNA by Southern blotting. ***c*** Time-course experiment. A homogenous pool of purified virus was made from gradient fraction #6, #7 and #8 and distributed among three culture dishes of primary tupaia hepatocytes. The cells were harvested on days 1, 7 and 16 post-infection. RC = Relaxed circular DNA; CCC = covalenty closed circular DNA; SS = single-stranded DNA. The cccDNA signal is equivalent to about 10^6 HBV genomes.

Figure 2c shows a time-course analysis, in which primary tupaia hepatocytes were harvested on days 1, 7 and 16 after infection with gradient-purified HBV. The viral DNA visible on day 1 is derived from attached particles harboring relaxed circular DNA (rcDNA). The most prominent DNA species detectable on day 7 is covalently closed circular DNA (cccDNA). Newly synthesized single-stranded DNA (ssDNA) is seen on day 16 post-infection. Only a minor fraction of viral particles succeeds in establishing infection and the total amount of viral DNA hardly increases from day 7 to day 16. In this respect, tupaia cells behave different from primary duck hepatocytes, where significant duck hepatitis B virus (DHBV) amplification takes place within the first week of infection [10]. The surface coding DNA sequence from inoculating HBV is identical to the corresponding RNA sequence derived from infected tupaia hepatocytes (data not shown). Therefore, selection of an infectious viral subpopulation does not seem to occur.

HBsAg and HBeAg secretion from HBV-infected tupaia hepatocytes is first detectable from day 6 on and increases up to day 12, when it reaches a plateau phase (fig. 3a). Measuring these antigens in culture supernatant represents a very convenient and sensitive assay to evaluate infection experiments. For purification of virus we also used sucrose, a gradient medium which results in good separation of HBV from subviral particles and plasma proteins [11]. Furthermore, polyethylene glycol (PEG), which was applied to enhance viral infectivity in primary human hepatocytes [2], was assessed for its effect on HBV infection of tupaia hepatocytes. The limitation of using serum for infection was indeed overcome by purification of viral particles on sucrose gradient or by adding 4% PEG to the cell-culture medium (fig. 3b). However, combining both procedures did not further enhance infection levels significantly (fig. 3c).

The specificity of the viral attachment and uptake leading to infection was verified by using monoclonal antibodies against the three HBV surface proteins. Especially the preS1 domain of LHBs, which is preferentially localized on the surface of HBV particles [12], is thought to play an important role during attachment to hepatocyte receptors [13, 14]. Furthermore, antibodies raised against a preS1 peptide (amino acid 21–47) are able to neutralize HBV infection in chimpanzees [15]. Preincubation of whole serum or isolated HBV virions with an excess of preS1 monoclonal antibody MA18/7 recognizing amino acid 20–23 of preS1 (genotype D) inhibited HBV infection of primary tupaia hepatocytes completely (fig. 3b).

The neutralizing capacity of preS2- and S-specific monoclonal antibodies varied. Only a conformational dependent S-specific antibody could completely inhibit infection of tupaia hepatocytes, but not a monoclonal antibody recognizing a linear S-epitope. Furthermore, none of the preS2-specific monoclonal antibodies tested was able to inhibit infection completely [16]. These results support the implication that HBV uses homologous preS1-dependent receptor systems on human cells and tupaia cells.

Using purified subviral particles, more than 70% of the primary tupaia hepatocytes were capable of binding preS1-rich HBsAg as detected by immuncytochemistry (fig. 4a). This binding could be inhibited by preincubating the particles with an excess of polyclonal anti-HBs generated by immunization with plasma-derived purified subviral particles (fig. 4b). The bound HBsAg was not

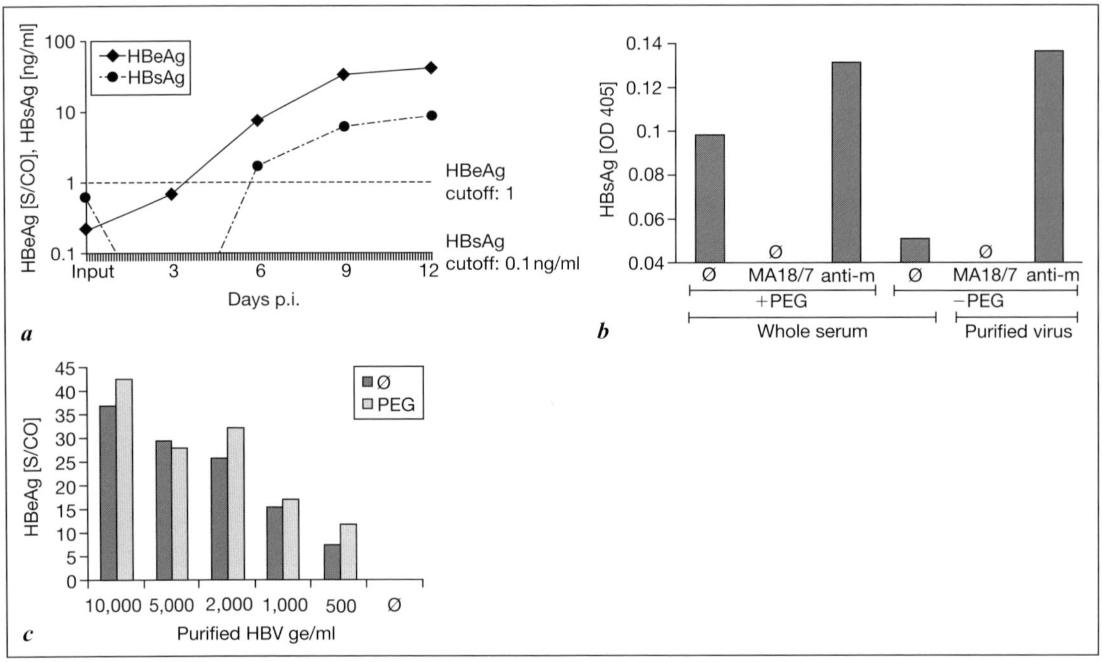

Fig. 3. ***a*** Time course of HBeAg and HBsAg secretion. The medium was changed every 3 days. Each dot represents HBeAg or HBsAg in the supernatant newly synthesized within 3 days. The dotted lines indicate the cutoffs for HBeAg (multiples of cutoff signal) and for HBsAg (0.1 ng/ml). S/CO, sample to cutoff signal. ***b*** Effect of PEG, sucrose gradient purification and monoclonal antibodies on viral infection levels. Confluent 5-cm dishes were inoculated with 180 μl of highly HBV-positive human serum (2×10^9 genome equivalents HBV/ml) diluted in medium. Inoculation was done in the presence of 4% PEG in the medium as indicated. After incubation overnight at 37°C in an incubator, viral input was removed; the plates were extensively washed and further incubated for 12 days at 37°C with medium refreshed every 3 days. HBsAg secretion was determined by an 'in-house' ELISA (OD 405) after 12 days. For specific inhibition of infection, whole serum or purified virions in infection medium were incubated with an excess of preS1-specific monoclonal antibody MA18/7 or with an irrelevant antibody (anti-mouse) prior to incubation with the cells. ***c*** Effect of polyethylene on infectivity of purified HBV. 24-well plates were infected with defined concentrations of sucrose-purified virus either in the presence of 4% PEG in the medium or without (Ø) and processed as described above. After 12 days, HBeAg in the supernatant was determined by ELISA.

evenly distributed on tupaia hepatocytes membranes, but localized to distinct membrane spots (fig. 4c, arrows). Very often, these areas are associated with special membrane structures like microvilli or lamellipodi. One might speculate that these structures are enriched in HBV receptors, since the sinusoidal side of hepatocytes in the liver is also heavily covered with microvilli [17]. A large

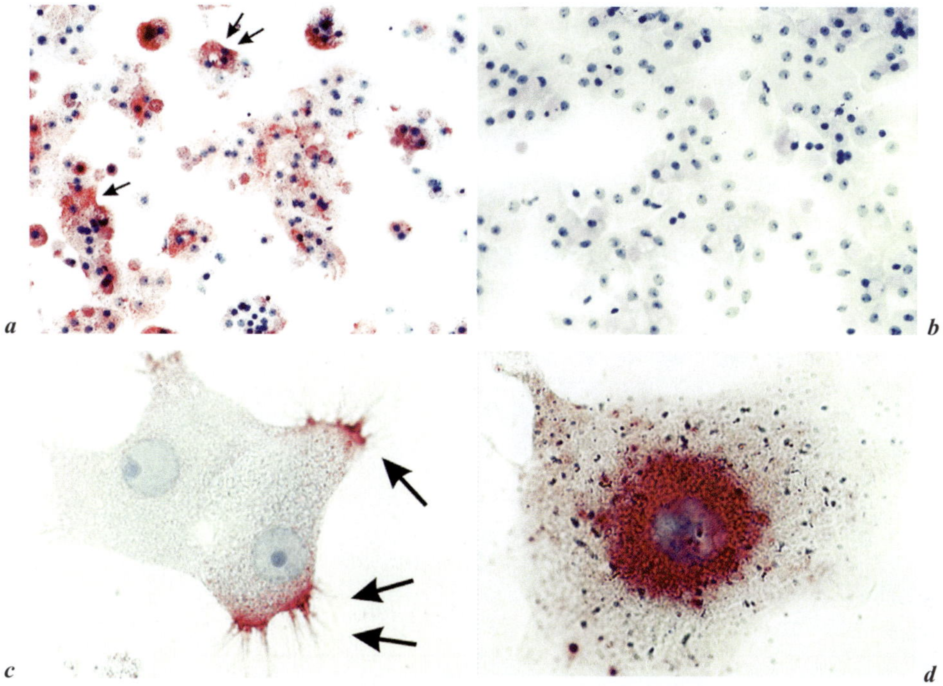

Fig. 4. Binding and uptake of subviral HBsAg particles. Immune staining of tupaia hepatocytes after incubation with purified LHBs-rich HBV subviral particles for 1 h at 37°C with antibodies against the S domain (red) and counterstained with Meyer's hemalaun (blue). Binding of HBsAg particles to primary tupaia hepatocytes is detected as seen (***a***) (magn. ×100), but not after preincubation of the inoculum with polyclonal anti-HBs antibodies (***b***). At higher magnification (×400) HBs particles are detected at distinct areas of the plasma membrane (***c***). Some hepatocytes show a pattern suggesting uptake of HBsAg (***d***).

portion of the cells showed signs of HBsAg uptake and subsequent transport to a yet undefined perinuclear region (fig. 4d). Within 2 h, this staining strongly decreases, which may be due to destruction of the HBsAg conformational epitope in an endosomal or lysosomal compartment.

Recently a novel hepadnavirus has been discovered in blood samples from woolly monkeys, a primate species endemic in South America. The woolly monkey hepatitis B virus (WMHBV) represents a pathogenic agent endogenous to woolly monkey and is closely related to the human virus [18]. Interestingly, primary tupaia hepatocytes are also susceptible to WMHBV. Similar to human HBV, the infection levels are low with non-processed serum but are significantly enhanced when gradient-purified WMHBV particles are applied (fig. 5a). In addition to cccDNA, the newly formed ssDNA as well as rcDNA are clearly

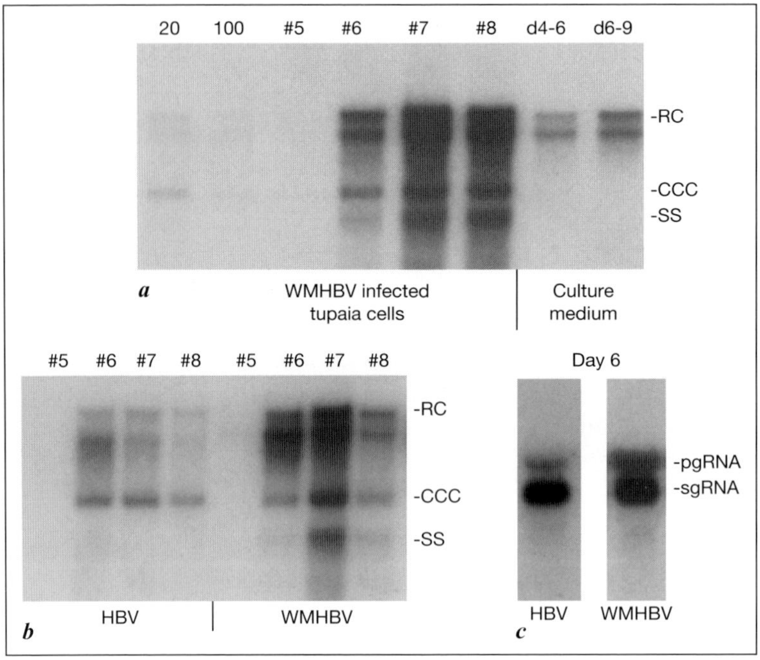

Fig. 5. ***a*** Infection with woolly monkey hepatitis B virus. Primary tupaia hepatocytes were infected with 20 and 100 μl of WMHBV-positive woolly monkey serum or with fractions #5, #6, #7 and #8 from a Nycodenz gradient loaded with 200 μl of WMHBV-positive serum (10^9 genomes/ml). The culture supernatants from days 4–6 and days 6–9 were collected. The hepatocytes were harvested on day 9 post-infection. Viral DNA was prepared from cells and culture medium, respectively, and visualized by Southern blotting. ***b*** Comparison of HBV and WMHBV infection. Primary tupaia hepatocytes were infected with equal amounts of purified HBV or WMHBV in a side-by-side approach. The cells were harvested on day 6 post-infection and analyzed for viral DNA by Southern blotting. ***c*** Viral transcripts in HBV- and WMHBV-infected tupaia hepatocytes. The cells were infected with purified HBV or WMHBV and harvested on day 6 post-infection. Total RNA was extracted and analyzed by Northern blotting. pgRNA = Pregenomic RNA; sgRNA = subgenomic RNA.

detectable in WMHBV-infected cells and viral particles are secreted into culture supernatant.

The WMHBV replication rate in primary tupaia hepatocytes is higher than the HBV replication rate and newly formed ssDNA is seen already on day 6 post-infection, whereas it is absent at the corresponding time point in the HBV-infected cells (fig. 5b). As shown in figure 5c, slightly more pregenomic RNA (pgRNA) relative to subgenomic RNA (sgRNA) is formed in WMHBV-infected cells than in HBV-infected cells, which may account for the divergent replication rates of the respective viruses. Compatible to this observation, there are significant differences in the core promoter sequences of the WMHBV and HBV genome. So far, we have not tested whether human hepatocytes are susceptible to WMHBV infection and it remains to be determined whether the replication rates of HBV and WMHBV also differ in human cells.

The biochemical nature of the inhibitory serum component is not yet definitively clear. Based on the results obtained with blood samples from HBV-negative, non-vaccinated individuals, the inhibitory effect is not caused by surface-specific antibodies or empty subviral particles. According to preliminary results, equilibrium density gradient centrifugation of human serum results in an accumulation of inhibitory activity in the fractions between albumin and high-density lipoprotein (data not shown). Among other proteins, the corresponding gradient fractions contain the β_2-glycoprotein, also called apolipoprotein H because of its association with acidic phospholipids. Unfortunately, further purification attempts failed as the inhibitory activity got lost after gel filtration or ion exchange chromatography.

Interestingly, a specific interaction of β_2-glycoprotein with HBV has been described in former studies and the β_2-glycoprotein has been proposed to target HBV to the liver cells [19, 20]. However, our results argue against this hypothesis since β_2-glycoprotein and infectious particles were separated from each other during gradient sedimentation (data not shown). Therefore, instead of mediating virus-cell contact, the β_2-glycoprotein may actually hinder HBV from getting in touch with the hepatocyte.

The physiological function of β_2-glycoprotein is not yet finally determined. Complexes formed by β_2-glycoprotein and phospholipids act as an antigen in autoimmune disorders characterized by clinical events of recurrent thrombosis, indicating an involvement of β_2-glycoprotein in hemostasis [21]. The inhibitory effect of β_2-glycoprotein during in vitro infection might play only a minor role during natural infection in living humans because circulating blood is different from serum in respect to the various biochemical modifications of serum proteins taking place in the course of blood coagulation.

Compared to human cells, primary hepatocytes from *T. belangeri* have the principal advantage of being available from in-house-bred animals which allows for systematic investigations using cells prepared on experimental demand. Furthermore, the quality of the tupaia cells is quite reproducible, while the suitability of primary hepatocytes from human liver has been reported to be highly variable [22]. In contrast to the recently described hepatoma-derived cell line HepaRG [23], which becomes susceptible to HBV infection upon differentiation to a hepatocyte-like phenotype, primary tupaia hepatocytes do not need to be supplemented with dimethyl sulfoxide (DMSO).

In the current state the tupaia system is particularly well suited to screen antiviral drugs or HBV-specific antibodies for their inhibitory activity on infection [16, 24]. In addition, the tupaia cells may be used to search for agents which promote the elimination of cccDNA. More recently we succeeded in infecting tupaia hepatocytes with recombinant virions generated in transfected hepatoma cells (data not shown). Therefore, primary hepatocytes from *T. belangeri* will also allow for testing the infectivity of mutant HBV particles.

References

1 Gripon P, Diot C, Theze N, Fourel I, Loreal O, Brechot C, Guguen-Guillouzo C: Hepatitis B virus infection of adult human hepatocytes cultured in the presence of dimethyl sulfoxide. J Virol 1988;62:4136–4143.

2 Gripon P, Diot C, Guguen-Guillouzo C: Reproducible high level infection of cultured adult human hepatocytes by hepatitis B virus: Effect of polyethylene glycol on adsorption and penetration. Virology 1993;192:534–540.

3 Novacek MJ: Mammalian phylogeny: Shaking the tree. Nature 1992;356:121–125.

4 Schmitz J, Ohme M, Zischler H: The complete mitochondrial genome of *Tupaia belangeri* and the phylogenetic affiliation of scandentia to other eutherian orders. Mol Biol Evol 2000;17: 1334–1343.

5 Fuchs E, Schumacher M: Psychosocial stress affects pineal function in the tree shrew (*Tupaia belangeri*). Physiol Behav 1990;47:713–717.

6 Walter E, Keist R, Niederost B, Pult I, Blum HE: Hepatitis B virus infection of tupaia hepatocytes in vitro and in vivo. Hepatology 1996;24:1–5.

7 Yan RQ, Su JJ, Huang DR, Gan YC, Yang C, Huang GH: Human hepatitis B virus and hepatocellular carcinoma. I. Experimental infection of tree shrews with hepatitis B virus. J Cancer Res Clin Oncol 1996;122:283–288.

8 Kock J, Nassal M, MacNelly S, Baumert TF, Blum HE, von Weizsacker F: Efficient infection of primary tupaia hepatocytes with purified human and woolly monkey hepatitis B virus. J Virol 2001;75:5084–5049.

9 Fowler E, Raab-Traub N, Hester S: Purification of biologically active Epstein-Barr virus by affinity chromatography and non-ionic density gradient centrifugation. J Virol Methods 1985;11: 59–74.

10 Tuttleman JS, Pugh JC, Summers JW: In vitro experimental infection of primary duck hepatocyte cultures with duck hepatitis B virus. J Virol 1986;58:17–25.

11 Glebe D, Gerlich WH: Study of the endocytosis and intracellular localization of subviral particles of hepatitis B virus in primary hepatocytes. Methods Mol Med 2004;96:143–152.

12 Heermann KH, Goldmann U, Schwartz W, Seyffarth T, Baumgarten H, Gerlich WH: Large surface proteins of hepatitis B virus containing the pre-S sequence. J Virol 1984;52:396–402.

13 Pontisso P, Ruvoletto MG, Gerlich WH, Heermann KH, Bardini R, Alberti A: Identification of an attachment site for human liver plasma membranes on hepatitis B virus particles. Virology 1989; 173:522–530.

14 Le Seyec J, Chouteau P, Cannie I, Guguen-Guillouzo C, Gripon P: Infection process of the hepatitis B virus depends on the presence of a defined sequence in the pre-S1 domain. J Virol 1999;73:2052–2057.

15 Neurath AR, Seto B, Strick N: Antibodies to synthetic peptides from the preS1 region of the hepatitis B virus (HBV) envelope (env) protein are virus-neutralizing and protective. Vaccine 1989;7:234–236.

16 Glebe D, Aliakbari M, Krass P, Knoop EV, Valerius KP, Gerlich WH: Pre-S1 antigen-dependent infection of tupaia hepatocyte cultures with human hepatitis B virus. J Virol 2003;77:9511–9521.

17 Phillips MJ: Biology and pathobiology of actin in the liver; in Arias IM, Boyer JL, Fausto N, Jakoby WB, Shafritz DA (eds): The Liver: Biology and Pathobiology. New York, Raven Press, 1994, pp 19–32.

18 Lanford RE, Chavez D, Brasky KM, Burns RB, Rico-Hesse R: Isolation of a hepadnavirus from the woolly monkey, a New World primate. Proc Natl Acad Sci USA 1998;95:5757–5761.
19 Mehdi H, Kaplan MJ, Anlar FY, Yang X, Bayer R, Sutherland K, Peeples ME: Hepatitis B virus surface antigen binds to apolipoprotein H. J Virol 1994;68:2415–2424.
20 Stefas I, Rucheton M, D'Angeac AD, Morel-Baccard C, Seigneurin JM, Zarski JP, Martin M, Cerutti M, Bossy JP, Misse D, Graafland H, Veas F: Hepatitis B virus Dane particles bind to human plasma apolipoprotein H. Hepatology 2001;33:207–217.
21 Rand JH: Molecular pathogenesis of the antiphospholipid syndrome. Circ Res 2002;90:29–37.
22 Galle P, Hagelstein RJ, Kommerell B, Volkmann M, Schranz P, Zentgraf H: In vitro experimental infection of primary human hepatocytes with hepatitis B virus. Gastroenterology 1994; 106:664–673.
23 Gripon P, Rumin S, Urban S, Le Seyec J, Glaise D, Cannie I, Guyomard C, Lucas J, Trepo C, Guguen-Guillouzo C: Infection of a human hepatoma cell line by hepatitis B virus. Proc Natl Acad Sci USA 2002;99:15655–15660.
24 Kock J, Baumert TF, Delaney WE, Blum HE, von Weizsacker F: Inhibitory effect of adefovir and lamivudine on the initiation of hepatitis B virus infection in primary tupaia hepatocytes. Hepatology 2003;38:1410–1418.
25 Von Weizsacker F, Kock J, MacNelly S, Ren S, Blum HE, Nassal M: The tupaia model for the study of hepatitis B virus: Direct infection and HBV genome transduction of primary tupaia hepatocytes. Methods Mol Med 2004;96:153–62.

Josef Köck
Department of Medicine II, Hugstetter Strasse 55
DE–79106 Freiburg (Germany)
Tel. +49 761 2703758, Fax +49 761 2703372, E-Mail josefkoeck@web.de

von Weizsäcker F, Roggendorf M (eds): Models of Viral Hepatitis.
Monogr Virol. Basel, Karger, 2005, vol 25, pp 106–118

Tupaia belangeri as a Model for Hepatitis C Virus Infection

Thomas F. Baumert, Heidi Barth, Xiping Zhao, Peter Schürmann, Zhen-Ya Tang, Mohammed I. Adah, Hubert E. Blum, Fritz von Weizsäcker

Department of Medicine II, University of Freiburg, Freiburg, Germany

Hepatitis C virus (HCV) is a major cause of post-transfusion and community-acquired hepatitis in the world [1–4]. The majority of HCV-infected individuals develop chronic hepatitis that may progress to liver cirrhosis and hepatocellular carcinoma [5]. Treatment options for chronic HCV infection are limited and a vaccine to prevent HCV infection is not available [5–7]. The lack of an in vitro cell culture model for efficient propagation of HCV virions has hampered biological and physiochemical studies on the virion and its mechanism of cell entry and infection. Furthermore, the lack of a convenient small animal model impedes the study of HCV pathogenesis as well as the development and preclinical evaluation of antiviral therapeutics and vaccines. In this chapter we will review recent studies evaluating *Tupaia belangeri* as a model for the study of HCV infection.

HCV has been classified in a separate genus (*Hepacivirus*) of the Flaviviridae family. The virion contains a positive-stranded RNA genome of approximately 9.6 kilobases [3]. The genome consists of a highly conserved 5′ non-coding region followed by a long open reading frame of 9,030–9,099 nucleotides that is translated into a single polyprotein of 3,010–3,030 amino acids. Processing of the polyprotein occurs by a combination of host and viral proteases. The HCV structural proteins comprise the putative nucleocapsid or core protein (C) and the two envelope glycoproteins E1 and E2 [3]. The non-structural proteins NS2, NS3, NS4A, NS4B, NS5A, and NS5B are required for viral protein processing and replication [8, 9]. Viral replication occurs via a negative-strand RNA intermediate. The non-structural proteins form a multi-protein complex that, in analogy to other positive-strand RNA viruses, is

Table 1. HCV research models [modified from 4]

Model system	Application	Reference
In vitro model systems		
Subgenomic and full-length HCV replicons	Analysis of HCV replication and screening of antiviral agents	9
Virus-like particles and retroviral HCV pseudoparticles	Analysis of virus-cell interaction	19, 21, 30
Primary hepatocytes (human, tupaia), human biliary epithelial cells, human lymphocytic cell lines	Analysis of virus-cell interaction, early steps of infection, virus neutralization	12, 43, 45, 59, 72, 73
Animal models		
Chimpanzee	Natural history of infection and disease/Clinical, virologic and immunologic studies/ Vaccination, treatment and rechallenge studies	74–76
Tupaia belangeri	Analysis of transient infection	58
Urokinase plasminogen activator (uPA)-transgenic HCV infection mice transplanted with human hepatocytes	Screening of antibodies and antiviral agents	48

associated with intracellular membranes [10]. HCV preferentially replicates in the cytoplasm of hepatocytes but distinct HCV sequences have also been isolated from dendritic cells [11] and viral replication has been demonstrated in B cells [12]. A special feature of HCV replication is the rapid generation of virus variants. Based on the genomic variability in a small region of NS5B, HCV has been classified in six major genotypes and 100 subtypes worldwide [3]. Furthermore, several distinct but closely related HCV sequences coexist within each infected individual. These are referred to as quasispecies and reflect the high replication rate of the virus and the lack of a proofreading capacity of the RNA-dependent RNA polymerase [13].

Due to the lack of a small animal model and efficient cell culture systems for HCV infection, alternative models have been developed to gain important information on the putative HCV life cycle (table 1). These models include virus-like and pseudotype particles to characterize interactions between viral and host cell compounds and HCV replicons to study viral replication.

Current HCV Model Systems and Their Limitations

In vitro Model Systems

The first step in the initiation of a virus infection is the attachment of the virion to the host cell, which is usually determined by an interaction between viral surface glycoproteins and specific cell-surface-receptor(s). In the absence of native virions, virus-like particles (VLPs) generated in insect cells have been successfully used as a surrogate model to study the host cell membrane interaction of several viruses [14–17]. Several laboratories, including ours, have demonstrated that the HCV structural proteins assemble into enveloped VLPs with morphologic, biophysical, and antigenic properties similar to putative virions from infected humans [18–29]. In contrast to individually expressed envelope glycoproteins, the E1–E2 heterodimers of insect cell-derived HCV-like particles (HCV-LPs) are presumably presented in a native, virion-like conformation [18–26]. Similar to virions, HCV-LPs bind and enter hepatoma and lymphoma cell lines [19, 23]. An alternative approach to study viral entry is the model system of retroviral HCV pseudoparticles containing functional E1–E2 envelope protein complexes [30–32]. Similar to HCV-LPs, HCV pseudoparticles enter human hepatocytes and defined hepatoma cells [30–32]. These model systems allowed to study the functional role of several cell surface proteins – including the tetraspanin CD81 [30, 33], the LDL receptor [34], the scavenger receptor B1 [30, 35], DC-SIGN [36] and highly sulfated heparan sulfate [19] – for envelope-cell surface interaction. However, since binding and entry of HCV-LPs and HCV pseudoparticles does not result in a productive infection, it is still unclear whether any of these molecules is sufficient to mediate initiation of HCV infection.

A breakthrough for the study of replication and definition of the components of the viral replication complex has been the development of HCV replicons, based on the self-replication of engineered minigenomes in human hepatoma cell lines [9, 10, 37–40]. Replicon-based systems have allowed to elucidate and dissect the viral replication complex, study mechanisms of viral resistance and explore novel antiviral approaches (see chapter by V. Lohmann et al.). Although extremely useful in the study of HCV genomic replication and screening for antiviral drugs, this system does not yet allow the study of viral infection or virus particle production [38].

Several in vitro models for the study of HCV infection have been proposed: These models include human lymphocytic cell lines [12, 41, 42], human biliary epithelial cells [43], and primary hepatocytes from humans [44, 45] or chimpanzees [46]. Limitations of these models are the very low level of HCV replication requiring the use of ultrasensitive nested RT/PCR methods for detection and the variable quality of host cells such as human hepatocytes obtained from surgical specimens.

Animal Models

The chimpanzee (*Pan troglodytes*) is the only non-human host serving as an in vivo model for HCV infection [47]. Although chimpanzees are easily infected with HCV and develop acute or chronic hepatitis, these animals are rare and require a high cost of maintenance.

Efforts at establishing small animal models for HCV infection have now made progress by the development of a mouse model containing a chimeric liver of mouse and human hepatocytes [48]. By transplantation of human hepatocytes to newborn immunodeficient homozygous Alb-uPA mice, the Alb-uPA mouse liver will be partially repopulated by human hepatocytes. The transplanted hepatocytes can be infected with serum from HCV-infected humans, resulting in HCV viremia lasting more than 10 weeks [48]. This model may allow the assessment of HCV infection in vivo and the study of new antiviral therapies. However, the use of this mouse model system for the study of HCV immunopathogenesis or vaccine research is limited by the lack of a functional immune system. Furthermore, technical difficulties in hepatocyte repopulation and survival of immunodeficient homozygous Alb-uPA limit this model for a convenient application and widespread use at the present time.

The tree shrew, *T. belangeri*, is a mammal that is endemic to subtropical areas of Southeast Asia [49]. *T. belangeri* has been shown to be susceptible to a variety of human viruses including herpes simplex, (HBV), and rotavirus [50–54]. Primary tupaia hepatocytes (PTH) can be efficiently infected with HBV [55–57] allowing the study of HBV entry and replication (see chapter by J. Köck and D. Glebe). Two studies have evaluated the use of *T. belangeri* as a model for HCV infection in vivo and in vitro [58, 59].

HCV Infection of T. belangeri *in vivo*

One study has demonstrated that *T. belangeri* can be infected in vivo with HCV [58]. Intravenous inoculation of tupaias using pooled HCV positive sera resulted in viremia and anti-HCV seroconversion in some of the inoculated animals. Transient or intermittent viremia occurred in 34.8% (8/23) of tupaias inoculated with HCV genotype 1b. The level of viremia was low (up to 3.5×10^5 copies/ml in serum). In another experimental approach using a subgroup of 4 animals, the authors examined the effect of whole-body irradiation (750 cGy) on HCV infection. Viremia lasted longer and anti-HCV antibodies tended to reach higher titers in irradiated as compared to non-irradiated animals. The authors concluded that radiation-induced immunosuppression may modify the course of infection. None of the inoculated animals developed chronic infection. A subgroup of the inoculated animals demonstrated significant ALT elevation, suggesting HCV-induced liver disease [58]. The ALT peak occurred in most of the animals between the 8th and 12th week following inoculation, similar to experimental HCV infection in chimpanzees [60]. Examination of liver biopsy specimens obtained from tupaias with elevated ALT levels and/or detectable anti-HCV antibody showed ballooning degeneration of hepatocytes, together with multinucleated liver cells and macrovesicular focal necrosis with inflammatory infiltrate [58]. However, some of these morphological alterations were also observed in control animals. The animals used for this study were captured in the wild and wild tupaias are known to be frequently infected by viruses, such as tree shrew herpes virus, which may cause spontaneous hepatitis. Therefore, the origin of the animals precludes the interpretation of these changes as solely due to HCV infection [58].

Our own experience with the in vivo infection of *T. belangeri* showed similar results: only a minority of animals inoculated with serum-derived HCV demonstrated evidence for successful infection as shown by transient detection of HCV RNA in serial serum samples (S. MacNelly, F. von Weizsäcker, unpubl. results).

Lack of chronic infection and infection in only some of the inoculated animals limit the use of tupaias for preclinical evaluation of antivirals and vaccines. The lack of a clear causal association between HCV infection and liver disease also preclude the use of this model for the study of HCV pathogenesis at the present time. Novel approaches for the establishment of a chronic infection and the efficient infection of all inoculated animals is required to use tupaia as an in vivo model for HCV infection.

Limited infection efficiency in tupaias in vivo may be the result of two factors: (1) Since *T. belangeri* does not represent the natural host for HCV infection, innate and adaptive antiviral immune responses of the infected animals may rapidly suppress and terminate viral infection, and (2) HCV derived from humans is not adapted for infection of tupaia hepatocytes. The latter hypothesis is supported by the observation that wooly monkey HBV – infecting a species more closely related to tupaias – replicates more efficiently in tupaia hepatocytes than human HBV [55]. To address the questions raised above, Zhao et al. [59] studied HCV infection of PTH. The model of primary hepatocytes allows the study of HCV infection in the absence of antiviral immune responses and is able to conveniently address the role of virus-specific factors for viral infection.

In vitro HCV Infection of Primary Tupaia Hepatocytes

PTH can be successfully infected by HCV using serum-derived HCV [59]. Incubation of PTH with serum or plasma from individuals chronically infected with HCV led to a time-dependent, de novo synthesis of positive-strand HCV RNA in hepatocytes. Due to the high sensitivity of PCR, it is most important to demonstrate that the RNA detected does not represent residual input HCV RNA. Besides time-course experiments, this question was specifically addressed by the detection of negative-strand HCV RNA, the analysis of quasispecies during infection and the detection of newly synthesized viral proteins [59]. Using a highly strand-specific RT/PCR method, newly synthesized negative-strand HCV RNA was detected in infected hepatocytes [59]. Newly synthesized positive-strand HCV RNA could be also detected in the culture medium. HCV RNA in hepatocytes and medium was resistant to ribonuclease treatment indicating the presence of packaged viral RNA, consistent with the presence of HCV virions. In addition, HCV protein synthesis in infected PTH could be demonstrated using immunofluorescence and high-titer anti-HCV antibodies present in human sera. Furthermore, the virus could be passaged from infected cells to naive hepatocytes. Successful viral passage was demonstrated by the detection of positive- and negative-strand HCV RNA in PTH [59]. The selection of certain variants and formation of new viral genomes during infection could be demonstrated by comparative analysis of viral quasispecies in inocula and infected hepatocytes. Analysis of HCV quasispecies in PTH infected with a well-characterized plasma from a chronically infected HCV patient [61–65] revealed a selection for HCV variants in the hypervariable region 1 of the E2 region consisting of H77 consensus sequence [63]. These data suggest that clones of H77C consensus recently shown to be infectious in chimpanzees also have the ability to infect PTH [63]. Following viral passage, a defined minority population containing a novel HVR-1 mutation emerged. These data confirmed infection of hepatocytes with passaged virus and are consistent with recent longitudinal analyses of H77 quasispecies evolution in man and chimpanzees demonstrating time-dependent development of new mutations [64, 65].

Both virus- and host-specific factors may be important for successful HCV infection in tupaias in vitro and in vivo. Infection of hepatocytes was dependent on defined inocula and required a minimal infectious dose [59]. Since only one inoculum (H77 7-12-77) was tested for infectivity in chimpanzees, it is not known whether infectivity of tupaia hepatocytes correlates with infectivity in chimpanzees. Infectivity of HCV serum samples was not associated with genotype or HCV antibody profile [59]. There was no correlation between the absence or presence of antibodies against the envelope proteins and infectivity [59]. These data suggest that only certain HCV isolates have the ability to infect and replicate efficiently in tupaia hepatocytes. This hypothesis would be in line with recent studies resulting in the isolation of infectious full-length or replication-competent subgenomic HCV RNAs. These studies have elegantly demonstrated that specific HCV RNAs are either infectious in vivo or are able to replicate efficiently in hepatoma cells. Adaptive mutations appear to play a key role overcoming these restrictions [9, 39]. Isolate-specific viral factors required for PTH infection may include a defined virus envelope protein structure allowing efficient viral entry into PTH or defined structural or regulatory features of the viral replicative complex allowing efficient viral replication. This hypothesis is corroborated by the results of viral quasispecies analysis in infected cells demonstrating a selection of defined variants and the suppression of others following viral infection. Further characterization of the infectious isolates may allow to define tupaia-tropic inocula. The detailed analysis of intracellular HCV RNA after successful infection and passage may ultimately result in the isolation of full-length HCV RNA efficiently replicating in PTH. Studies analyzing potentially adaptive mutations in the HCV genome required for infection of PTH are under way.

Interestingly, very recent studies have indicated that the purification of virions by gradient centrifugation enhances the infection efficiency of serum-derived HCV (P. Schürmann, T. Baumert, unpubl. observations). This observation suggests that – similar to previous findings described for HBV infection of tupaia hepatocytes [55] – human serum may contain a factor inhibiting HCV infection. Further studies are under way to study this factor in detail.

Following the detailed characterization of viral infection of PTH, it is critical to explore whether this model system can be applied to study important features of the HCV life cycle. Levels of HCV replication in tupaia hepatocytes are approx. 100- to 10,000-fold lower than levels of viral replication in replicon systems. In contrast to convenient detection of viral replication and protein synthesis by Northern and Western blots in replicon systems, ultrasensitive methods such as RT-PCR are required to assess viral replication in primary hepatocytes. This difference clearly demonstrates that the replicon system is the model of choice for the study of viral replication, antiviral drug screening and study of antiviral resistance. However, in contrast to replicon systems, the tupaia model system allows the study of early steps of viral infection such as virus-cell surface interaction, viral entry and initiation of viral infection.

The successful application of the tupaia hepatocyte model system for the study of early steps of viral infection has been demonstrated by studying the functional role of HCV receptor candidates CD81 and SR-B1 for the initiation of viral infection of hepatocytes [59, 66]. Pileri and colleagues [33, 67] reported that HCV E2 could specifically bind to cell surface molecule CD81 expressed on lymphoma cells. CD81 is a member of the tetraspanin family, and has been shown to play an important role in signal transduction and adhesion in the immune system [68]. To assess whether viral entry in tupaia hepatocytes was CD81-dependent, tupaia CD81 was identified and characterized. Tupaia and human CD81 exhibited a high degree of homology at the amino acid level in the E2-binding domain of CD81 [59]. This finding is consistent with the genetic relationship between the two species. Furthermore, monoclonal anti-human CD81 antibodies showed strong binding to tupaia CD81 in immunoblot and flow cytometry. Analysis of the interaction of HCV E2 glycoprotein with tupaia hepatocytes using FACS demonstrated that recombinant HCV E2 protein could bind to freshly isolated tupaia hepatocytes. Cellular binding of E2 to PTH was dose-dependent and saturable and exhibited a similar binding profile as recently described for human hepatoma cells [23, 59, 67]. Although anti-CD81 antibodies used in this study interact strongly with tupaia CD81, and have previously been shown to inhibit the interaction of E2 with CD81 [67, 69, 70], these antibodies failed to inhibit binding of E2 to tupaia hepatocytes under CD81-saturating conditions. Furthermore, soluble CD81 did not block E2 binding at concentrations shown to inhibit E2 binding to Molt-4 lymphoma cells. The finding of CD81-independent E2-hepatocyte interaction implied that HCV infection of tupaia hepatocytes may be mediated by additional or other molecules besides CD81. This hypothesis was confirmed in experiments analyzing HCV infection of PTH in the presence of anti-CD81 antibodies or a soluble fusion protein containing the CD81 large extracellular loop. Neither monoclonal anti-human CD81 antibodies binding to tupaia CD81 nor soluble CD81 were able to block viral infection of tupaia hepatocytes. This finding clearly demonstrates that viral infection requires additional or other receptors besides CD81. This observation is corroborated by recent observations providing indirect evidence for the lack of CD81 as a receptor mediating viral entry: (1) the molecule is expressed ubiquitously on the surface of various cell types not limited to HCV susceptible cells [68]; (2) binding of sucrose gradient-purified virions from HCV-infected individuals to lymphoma cells and foreskin fibroblasts does not require HCV-CD81-interaction [71], and (3) cellular binding of HCV-LPs and entry of retroviral HCV pseudotype particles requires other or additional liver-specific co-factor(s) besides CD81 [21, 23, 30].

The human scavenger receptor class B type 1 (SR-B1) represents a novel HCV receptor candidate mediating cellular binding of recombinant HCV glycoprotein E2 to human HepG2 hepatoma cells [35]. A recent study analyzed the functional role of SR-B1 for HCV infection of PTH [66]. Sequence analysis of cloned SR-B1 cDNA revealed a high degree of homology (88%) between human and tupaia SR-B1. Using flow cytometry and polyclonal anti-human and tupaia SR-B1 antibodies (generated by genetic immunization of mice), SR-B1 was detected on the cell surface of PTH. Western blotting indicated a similar size of SR-B1 in PTH and human HepG2 cells (80–85 kDa). Recombinant E2 and HCV-LPs demonstrated a dose-dependent and saturable binding to PTH as shown by flow cytometry. Incubation of PTH with anti-human or anti-tupaia SR-B1 antibodies resulted in a marked and dose-dependent inhibition of cellular E2 binding. However, in vitro HCV infection of tupaia hepatocytes was not blocked by anti-SR-B1 antibodies suggesting that viral entry is mediated by SR-B1 in concert with additional cell surface molecules [66]. These findings are corroborated by other model systems demonstrating that entry of HCV pseudoparticles into human HuH-7 hepatoma cells [30] or cellular binding of HCV-LPs to HepG2 cells (H. Barth, T.F. Baumert, unpubl. observations) can only be partially inhibited by anti-SR B1 antibodies.

Taken together, these functional studies demonstrate that PTH represent a useful model system to study the functional role of HCV receptor candidates and early stages of the viral life cycle such as viral envelope-hepatocyte cell surface interaction and the initiation of infection.

Prospects for the Future

Future applications for the PTH model systems include the study of antibody-mediated neutralization and as well as the assessment of novel antivirals interfering with viral attachment or viral entry. The tupaia system is ideally suited to address these questions. More studies are needed to define viral (e.g., adaptive mutations) and host factors determining infection efficiency. The exploration of these factors may give novel insight into HCV biology and pathogenesis.

In vivo HCV infection of tupaia is transient, low-level and occurring in only some of the inoculated animals [58]. The findings in PTH suggest that the use of tupaia as an in vivo model could depend on the selection of tupaia-tropic HCV strains [59]. Serial passage of gradient purified HCV in PTH may select for suitable inocula for efficient in vivo infection. Furthermore, the exploration of viral and host factors determining infection efficiency in vitro and in vivo may ultimately allow the establishment of an urgently needed small animal model.

References

1 Choo QL, Kuo A, Weiner AJ, Overby LR, Bradley DW, Houghton M: Isolation of a cDNA clone derived from a blood-borne non-A, non-B viral hepatitis genome. Science 1989;244:359–362.
2 Lauer GM, Walker BD: Hepatitis C virus infection. N Engl J Med 2001;345:41–52.
3 Lindenbach BD, Rice CM: Flaviviridae: The viruses and their replication; in Knipe DM, Howley PM, Griffin DE, Lamb RA, Martin MA, Roizman B, Straus SE (eds): Fields Virology. Baltimore, Lippincott Williams & Wilkins, 2001, pp 991–1041.
4 Racanelli V, Rehermann B: Hepatitis C virus infection: When silence is deception. Trends Immunol 2003;24:456–464.
5 Hoofnagle JH: Course and outcome of hepatitis C. Hepatology 2002;36:S21–S29.
6 Inchauspe G, Feinstone S: Development of a hepatitis C virus vaccine. Clin Liver Dis 2003;7: 243–259.
7 Baumert TF, Lechmann M, Liang TJ: Novel strategies in hepatitis C virus vaccine development; in Rodes J (ed): Therapy in Hepatology. Barcelona, Medicina STM Editores, 2001, pp 345–357.
8 Bartenschlager R, Lohmann V: Replication of hepatitis C virus. J Gen Virol 2000;81:1631–1648.

9 Lohmann V, Körner F, Koch JO, Herian U, Theilmann L, Bartenschlager R: Replication of subgenomic hepatitis C virus RNAs in a hepatoma cell line. Science 1999;285:110–113.
10 Pietschmann T, Bartenschlager R: The hepatitis C virus replicon system and its application to molecular studies. Curr Opin Drug Discov Dev 2001;4:657–664.
11 Bain C, Fatmi A, Zoulim F, Zarski JP, Trepo C, Inchauspe G: Impaired allostimulatory function of dendritic cells in chronic hepatitis C infection. Gastroenterology 2001;120:512–524.
12 Sung VM, Shimodaira S, Doughty AL, Picchio GR, Can H, Yen TS, Lindsay KL, Levine AM, Lai MM: Establishment of B-cell lymphoma cell lines persistently infected with hepatitis C virus in vivo and in vitro: The apoptotic effects of virus infection. J Virol 2003;77:2134–2146.
13 Bukh J, Miller RH, Purcell RH: Biology and genetic heterogeneity of hepatitis C virus. Clin Exp Rheumatol 1995;13(suppl 13):3–7.
14 Tamura M, Natori K, Kobayashi M, Miyamura T, Takeda N: Interaction of recombinant Norwalk virus particles with the 105-kilodalton cellular binding protein, a candidate receptor molecule for virus attachment. J Virol 2000;74:11589–11597.
15 Combita AL, Touze A, Bousarghin L, Christensen ND, Coursaget P: Identification of two cross-neutralizing linear epitopes within the L1 major capsid protein of human papillomaviruses. J Virol 2002;76:6480–6486.
16 Gilbert JM, Greenberg HB: Cleavage of rhesus rotavirus VP4 after arginine-247 is essential for rotavirus-like particle-induced fusion from without. J Virol 1998;72:5323–5327.
17 Giroglou T, Florin L, Schafer F, Streeck RE, Sapp M: Human papillomavirus infection requires cell surface heparan sulfate. J Virol 2001;75:1565–1570.
18 Baumert TF, Ito S, Wong DT, Liang TJ: Hepatitis C virus structural proteins assemble into virus-like particles in insect cells. J Virol 1998;72:3827–3836.
19 Barth H, Schafer C, Adah MI, Zhang F, Linhardt RJ, Toyoda H, Kinoshita-Toyoda A, Toida T, van Kuppevelt TH, Depla E, Von Weizsäcker F, Blum HE, Baumert TF: Cellular binding of hepatitis C virus envelope glycoprotein E2 requires cell surface heparan sulfate. J Biol Chem 2003; 278:41003–41012.
20 Baumert TF, Vergalla J, Satoi J, Thomson M, Lechmann M, Herion D, Greenberg HB, Ito S, Liang TJ: Hepatitis C virus-like particles synthesized in insect cells as a potential vaccine candidate. Gastroenterology 1999;117:1397–1407.
21 Triyatni M, Saunier B, Maruvada P, Davis AR, Ulianich L, Heller T, Patel A, Kohn LD, Liang TJ: Interaction of hepatitis C virus-like particles and cells: A model system for studying viral binding and entry. J Virol 2002;76:9335–9344.
22 Triyatni M, Vergalla J, Davis AR, Hadlock KG, Foung SK, Liang TJ: Structural features of envelope proteins on hepatitis C virus-like particles as determined by anti-envelope monoclonal antibodies and CD81 binding. Virology 2002;298:124–132.
23 Wellnitz S, Klumpp B, Barth H, Ito S, Depla E, Dubuisson J, Blum HE, Baumert TF: Binding of hepatitis C virus-like particles derived from infectious clone H77C to defined human cell lines. J Virol 2002;76:1181–1193.
24 Clayton RF, Owsianka A, Aitken J, Graham S, Bhella D, Patel AH: Analysis of antigenicity and topology of E2 glycoprotein present on recombinant hepatitis C virus-like particles. J Virol 2002; 76:7672–7682.
25 Owsianka A, Clayton RF, Loomis-Price LD, McKeating JA, Patel AH: Functional analysis of hepatitis C virus E2 glycoproteins and virus-like particles reveals structural dissimilarities between different forms of E2. J Gen Virol 2001;82:1877–1883.
26 Xiang J, Wunschmann S, George SL, Klinzman D, Schmidt WN, LaBrecque DR, Stapleton JT: Recombinant hepatitis C virus-like particles expressed by baculovirus: Utility in cell binding and antibody detection assays. J Med Virol 2002;68:537–543.
27 Blanchard E, Brand D, Trassard S, Goudeau A, Roingeard P: Hepatitis C virus-like particle morphogenesis. J Virol 2002;76:4073–4079.
28 Ezelle HJ, Markovic D, Barber GN: Generation of hepatitis C virus-like particles by use of a recombinant vesicular stomatitis virus vector. J Virol 76:12325–12334.
29 Blanchard E, Hourioux C, Brand D, Ait-Goughoulte M, Moreau A, Trassard S, Sizaret PY, Dubois F, Roingeard P: Hepatitis C virus-like particle budding: Role of the core protein and importance of its Asp111. J Virol 2003;77:10131–10138.

30 Bartosch B, Vitelli A, Granier C, Goujon C, Dubuisson J, Pascale S, Scarselli E, Cortese R, Nicosia A, Cosset FL: Cell entry of hepatitis C virus requires a set of co-receptors that include the CD81 tetraspanin and the SR-B1 scavenger receptor. J Biol Chem 2003;278:41624–41630.

31 Bartosch B, Dubuisson J, Cosset FL: Infectious hepatitis C virus pseudo-particles containing functional E1–E2 envelope protein complexes. J Exp Med 2003;197:633–642.

32 Hsu M, Zhang J, Flint M, Logvinoff C, Cheng-Mayer C, Rice CM, McKeating JA: Hepatitis C virus glycoproteins mediate pH-dependent cell entry of pseudotyped retroviral particles. Proc Natl Acad Sci USA 2003;100:7271–7276.

33 Pileri P, Uematsu Y, Campagnoli S, Galli G, Falugi F, Petracca R, Weiner AJ, Houghton M, Rosa D, Grandi G, Abrignani S: Binding of hepatitis C virus to CD81. Science 1998;282:938–941.

34 Agnello V, Abel G, Elfahal M, Knight GB, Zhang QX: Hepatitis C virus and other flaviviridae viruses enter cells via low density lipoprotein receptor. Proc Natl Acad Sci USA 1999;96: 12766–12771.

35 Scarselli E, Ansuini H, Cerino R, Roccasecca RM, Acali S, Filocamo G, Traboni C, Nicosia A, Cortese R, Vitelli A: The human scavenger receptor class B type I is a novel candidate receptor for the hepatitis C virus. EMBO J 2002;21:5017–5025.

36 Pohlmann S, Zhang J, Baribaud F, Chen Z, Leslie GJ, Lin G, Granelli-Piperno A, Doms RW, Rice CM, McKeating JA: Hepatitis C virus glycoproteins interact with DC-SIGN and DC-SIGNR. J Virol 2003;77:4070–4080.

37 Blight KJ, Kolykhalov AA, Rice CM: Efficient initiation of HCV RNA replication in cell culture. Science 2000;290:1972–1975.

38 Pietschmann T, Lohmann V, Kaul A, Krieger N, Rinck G, Rutter G, Strand D, Bartenschlager R: Persistent and transient replication of full-length hepatitis C virus genomes in cell culture. J Virol 2002;76:4008–4021.

39 Lohmann V, Hoffmann S, Herian U, Penin F, Bartenschlager R: Viral and cellular determinants of hepatitis C virus RNA replication in cell culture. J Virol 2003;77:3007–3019.

40 Lohmann V, Korner F, Dobierzewska A, Bartenschlager R: Mutations in hepatitis C virus RNAs conferring cell culture adaptation. J Virol 2001;75:1437–1449.

41 Morsica G, Tambussi G, Sitia G, Novati R, Lazzarin A, Lopalco L, Mukenge S: Replication of hepatitis C virus in B lymphocytes (CD19+). Blood 1999;94:1138–1139.

42 Favre D, Berthillon P, Trepo C: Removal of cell-bound lipoproteins: A crucial step for the efficient infection of liver cells with hepatitis C virus in vitro. C R Acad Sci III 2001;324:1141–1148.

43 Bichr S, Rende-Fournier R, Vona G, Yamamoto AM, Depla E, Maertens G, Brechot C: Detection of neutralizing antibodies to hepatitis C virus using a biliary cell infection model. J Gen Virol 2002;83:1673–1678.

44 Founier C, Sureau C, Coste J, Ducos J, Pageaux G, Larrey D, Domergue J, Maurel P: In vitro infection of adult normal human hepatocytes in primary culture by hepatitis C virus. J Gen Virol 1998;79:2367–2374.

45 Castet V, Fournier C, Soulier A, Brillet R, Coste J, Larrey D, Dhumeaux D, Maurel P, Pawlotsky JM: Alpha-interferon inhibits hepatitis C virus replication in primary human hepatocytes infected in vitro. J Virol 2002;76:8189–8199.

46 Lanford RE, Sureau C, Jacob JR, White R, Fuerst TR: Demonstration of in vitro infection of chimpanzee hepatocytes with hepatitis C virus using strand-specific RT/PCR. Virology 1994; 202:606–614.

47 Bukh J, Forns X, Emerson SU, Purcell RH: Studies of hepatitis C virus in chimpanzees and their importance for vaccine development. Intervirology 2001;44:132–142.

48 Mercer DF, Schiller DE, Elliott JF, Douglas DN, Hao C, Rinfret A, Addison WR, Fischer KP, Churchill TA, Lakey JR, Tyrrell DL, Kneteman NM: Hepatitis C virus replication in mice with chimeric human livers. Nat Med 2001;7:927–933.

49 Novacek MJ: Mammalian phylogeny: Shaking the tree. Nature 1992;356:121–125.

50 Davis GL, Nelson DR, Reyes GR: Future options for the management of hepatitis C. Semin Liver Dis 1999;19:103–112.

51 Park US, Su JJ, Ban KC, Qin L, Lee EH, Lee YI: Mutations in the p53 tumor suppressor gene in tree shrew hepatocellular carcinoma associated with hepatitis B virus infection and intake of aflatoxin B1. Gene 2000;251:73–80.

52 Pang QF, Liu JC, Wan XB, Qiu FX, Xu AY: Experimental infection of adult *Tupaia belangeri yunalis* with human rotavirus. Chin Med J (Engl) 1983;96:85–94.
53 Walter E, Keist R, Niederöst B, Pult I, Blum HE: Hepatitis B virus infection of tupaia hepatocytes in vitro and in vivo. Hepatology 1996;24:1–5.
54 Yan RQ, Su JJ, Huang DR, Gan YC, Yang C, Huang GH: Human hepatitis B virus and hepatocellular carcinoma. I. Experimental infection of tree shrews with hepatitis B virus. J Cancer Res Clin Oncol 1996;122:283–288.
55 Köck J, Nassal M, MacNelly S, Baumert TF, Blum HE, von Weizsäcker F: Efficient infection of primary tupaia hepatocytes with human and woolly monkey hepatitis B virus. J Virol 2001;75: 5084–5089.
56 Glebe D, Aliakbari M, Krass P, Knoop EV, Valerius KP, Gerlich WH: Pre-s1 antigen-dependent infection of tupaia hepatocyte cultures with human hepatitis B virus. J Virol 2003;77:9511–9521.
57 Kock J, Baumert TF, Delaney WE, Blum HE, von Weizsäcker F: Inhibitory effect of adefovir and lamivudine on the initiation of hepatitis B virus infection in primary tupaia hepatocytes. Hepatology 2003;38:1410–1418.
58 Xie ZC, Riezu-Boj JI, Lasarte JJ, Guillen J, Su JH, Civeira MP, Prieto J: Transmission of hepatitis C virus infection to tree shrews. Virology 1998;244:513–520.
59 Zhao X, Tang ZY, Klumpp B, Wolff-Vorbeck G, Barth H, Levy S, von Weizsäcker F, Blum HE, Baumert TF: Primary hepatocytes of *Tupaia belangeri* as a potential model for hepatitis C virus infection. J Clin Invest 2002;109:221–232.
60 Farci P, Alter HJ, Wong D, Miller RH, Shih JW, Jett B, Purcell RH: A long-term study of hepatitis C virus replication in non-A, non-B hepatitis. N Engl J Med 1991;325:98–104.
61 Farci P, Alter HJ, Wong DC, Miller RH, Govindarajan S, Engle R, Shapiro M, Purcell RH: Prevention of hepatitis C virus infection in chimpanzees after antibody- mediated in vitro neutralization. Proc Natl Acad Sci USA 1994;91:7792–7796.
62 Kolykhalov AA, Agapov EV, Blight KJ, Mihalik K, Feinstone SM, Rice CM: Transmission of hepatitis C by intrahepatic inoculation with transcribed RNA. Science 1997;277:570–574.
63 Yanagi M, Purcell RH, Emerson SU, Bukh J: Transcripts from a single full-length cDNA clone of hepatitis C virus are infectious when directly transfected into the liver of a chimpanzee. Proc Natl Acad Sci USA 1997;94:8738–8743.
64 Ogata N, Alter HJ, Miller RH, Purcell RH: Nucleotide sequence and mutation rate of the H strain of hepatitis C virus. Proc Natl Acad Sci USA 1991;88:3392–3396.
65 Major ME, Mihalik K, Fernandez J, Seidman J, Kleiner D, Kolykhalov AA, Rice CM, Feinstone SM: Long-term follow-up of chimpanzees inoculated with the first infectious clone for hepatitis C virus. J Virol 1999;73:3317–3325.
66 Barth H, Raffaele C, Mirko A, Schürmann P, Adah MI, Gissler B, von Weizsäcker F, Blum HE, Vitelli A, Scarselli E, Baumert TF: Interaction of hepatitis C virus with scavenger receptor B1 of primary tupaia hepatocytes. Presentation P-50, 10th International Meeting on HCV and Related Viruses, Kyoto, Japan, December 2–6, 2003.
67 Flint M, Maidens CM, Loomis-Price LD, Shotton C, Dubuisson J, Monk P, Higginbottom A, Levy S, McKeating J: Characterization of hepatitis C virus E2 glycoprotein interaction with a putative cellular receptor CD81. J Virol 1999;73:6235–6244.
68 Levy S, Todd SC, Maecker HT: CD81 (TAPA-1): A molecule involved in signal transduction and cell adhesion in the immune system. Annu Rev Immunol 1998;16:89–109.
69 Higginbottom A, Quinn ER, Kuo CC, Flint M, Wilson LH, Bianchi E, Nicosia A, Monk PN, McKeating JA, Levy S: Identification of amino acid residues in CD81 critical for interaction with hepatitis C virus envelope glycoprotein E2. J Virol 2000;74:3642–3649.
70 Flint M, Dubuisson J, Maidens C, Harrop R, Guile GR, Borrow P, McKeating JA: Functional characterization of intracellular and secreted forms of a truncated hepatitis C virus E2 glycoprotein. J Virol 2000;74:702–709.
71 Wunschmann S, Medh JD, Klinzmann D, Schmidt WN, Stapleton JT: Characterization of hepatitis C virus (HCV) and HCV E2 interactions with CD81 and the low-density lipoprotein receptor. J Virol 2000;74:10055–10062.
72 Shimizu Y, Iwamoto A, Hijikata M, Purcell RH, Yoshikura H: Evidence for in vitro replication of hepatitis C virus genome in a human T-cell line. Proc Natl Acad Sci USA 1992;89:5477–5481.

73 Shimizu YK, Hijikata M, Iwamoto A, Alter HJ, Purcell RH, Yoshikura H: Neutralizing antibodies against hepatitis C virus and the emergence of neutralization escape mutant viruses. J Virol 1994;68:1494–1500.
74 Bassett SE, Guerra B, Brasky K, Miskovsky E, Houghton M, Klimpel GR, Lanford RE: Protective immune response to hepatitis C virus in chimpanzees rechallenged following clearance of primary infection. Hepatology 2001;33:1479–1487.
75 Major ME, Mihalik K, Puig M, Rehermann B, Nascimbeni M, Rice CM, Feinstone SM: Previously infected and recovered chimpanzees exhibit rapid responses that control hepatitis C virus replication upon rechallenge. J Virol 2002;76:6586–6595.
76 Nascimbeni M, Mizukoshi E, Bosmann M, Major ME, Mihalik K, Rice CM, Feinstone SM, Rehermann B: Kinetics of CD4+ and CD8+ memory T-cell responses during hepatitis C virus rechallenge of previously recovered chimpanzees. J Virol 2003;77:4781–4793.

PD Dr. Thomas F. Baumert
Department of Medicine II, University of Freiburg
Hugstetter Strasse 55, DE–79106 Freiburg (Germany)
Tel. +49 761 2703401, Fax +49 761 2703259
E-Mail tbaumert@ukl.uni-freiburg.de

von Weizsäcker F, Roggendorf M (eds): Models of Viral Hepatitis.
Monogr Virol. Basel, Karger, 2005, vol 25, pp 119–134

Primary Human Hepatocytes as an in vitro Model for Hepatitis B Virus Infection

Stephan Boehm[a], *Wolfgang E. Thasler*[c], *Thomas S. Weiss*[b], *Wolfgang Jilg*[a]

[a]Institute for Medical Microbiology and Hygiene, and [b]Center for Liver Cell Research, University of Regensburg, Regensburg, and [c]Department of Surgery, Klinikum Grosshadern, University of Munich, Munich, Germany

Hepatitis B virus (HBV) represents the prototypic member of the genus *Orthohepadnavirus* within the family *Hepadnaviridae*, which forms a group of small enveloped DNA viruses with the typical biological features of high species specificity and hepatotropism. Animal models used for in vivo and in vitro infection experiments have been established for the hepadnavirus species of the woodchuck, the ground squirrel and the duck [1]. In vitro infection models are essential for the experimental analysis of the first steps of the viral life cycle, including attachment, entry and uncoating, and in particular for studies of the underlying molecular interactions between viral particles and target cells. Critical biological properties of HBV for the establishment of an in vitro infection model are not only the species specificity and cell tropism of the virus but also the requirement of high-grade differentiation of target cells for efficient infection in vitro. Therefore, the currently available in vitro models for HBV infection are mainly based on primary hepatocyte cultures, in which target cells for HBV can be maintained in a differentiated state for several weeks [2].

Early studies in the 1970s have shown that chimpanzees and to a lesser extent other high-order primates are susceptible to experimental infection with HBV [3]. Since then, the chimpanzee model provided the opportunity to study HBV infection in vivo for more than 30 years. However, in contrast to the in vivo situation, infection experiments with cultured primary chimpanzee hepatocytes revealed a loss of susceptibility of these cells in vitro [4]. Moreover, mainly due to ethical considerations, primary chimpanzee hepatocytes are not routinely available [5]. Therefore, an in vitro infection model for HBV based on primary chimpanzee hepatocytes has not been used widely.

More recently, successful in vivo and in vitro infection of hepatocytes from Asian tree shrews (*Tupaia belangeri*) has been reported [6]. These small animals are non-rodent mammals, which are classified into the family Tupaiidae within the order Scandentia [7]. Infection of adult and newborn animals results in transient HBV replication followed by rapid viral clearance; therefore, it does not reflect the natural course of HBV infection in humans or chimpanzees. In contrast, in vitro infection of primary tupaia hepatocytes seems to resemble infection of human cells very closely [8, 9]. Based on this observation, primary tupaia hepatocytes have already become an important model for in vitro studies of HBV infection.

The use of primary human hepatocytes for in vitro infection experiments has been limited for many years due to difficulties in isolation and cultivation of these cells in a highly differentiated state, and also due to the low efficiency of HBV infection of these cells in vitro. Since during the last two decades major progress has been made in cell isolation and cultivation as well as infection conditions, an in vitro infection model for HBV based on primary human hepatocytes has become a tool for studies of the biology of this virus [10, 11]. However, major limitations of this model are the variability of hepatocyte preparations as well as the use of different infection protocols and different methods for the detection of viral replication in vitro. Therefore, further improvements can only be achieved by the standardization of infection and culture conditions and the introduction of quantitative analysis of different infection parameters.

Characterization of the Human in vitro Infection Model for HBV

Hepatocyte Donors and Cell Isolation Procedure

The major drawback of the human system in comparison to the tupaia model is the high variability of human cell preparations. Human hepatocyte preparations are most often obtained from normal liver tissue within surgical specimens from patients with primary or secondary malignant liver tumors whereas tupaia hepatocytes are usually recovered from young and healthy animals. Several factors may therefore influence the amount and quality of cultivable human hepatocytes, as age and gender of the patient as well as underlying disease and therapy used. Thus, when liver tissue from 5 patients with cirrhosis and impaired liver function was used, a viable cell preparation could only be obtained in 1 case [11]. Age, gender, type of malignant disease or the

Table 1. Reduction of cell yields due to antitumor chemotherapy

Hepatocyte donor	Age years	Gender	Duration of ischemia min	Duration of cell isolation procedure min	Cell yield per g liver tissue
Patients without antitumor chemotherapy					
Donor 1	75	Female	20	98	26.2×10^6
Donor 2	71	Male	17	61	14.7×10^6
Donor 3	55	Male	33	84	18.9×10^6
Donor 4	62	Female	16	85	14.8×10^6
Donor 5	69	Male	21	109	8.4×10^6
Mean	66		21	87	16.6×10^6
Patients with antitumor chemotherapy					
Donor 6	55	Female	25	104	11.2×10^6
Donor 7	65	Male	28	84	8.0×10^6
Donor 8	51	Male	17	78	7.3×10^6
Donor 9	53	Male	21	89	2.6×10^6
Donor 10	53	Male	35	93	5.7×10^6
Mean	55		25	90	7.0×10^6

surgical procedure used had no major effect on total cell yields after hepatocyte isolation [11]; however, treatment with antitumor chemotherapy prior to liver surgery significantly reduced cell yields in our group of liver cell donors (table 1). Furthermore, prolonged duration of ischemia and collagenase perfusion time during the cell isolation procedure are critical parameters with negative effects on quality of hepatocyte preparations. Therefore, the two-step collagenase perfusion based on the method described by Seglen [12] has become the standard technique for isolation of primary human as well as tupaia hepatocytes [9, 11].

Culture Conditions for Primary Hepatocytes

Successful in vitro infection of primary hepatocytes with HBV depends on a high grade of differentiation of the cultured cells. Important factors for maintenance of functional hepatocytes in culture are (1) the supplementation of culture medium with hormones like insulin, glucagon and hydrocortisone or dexamethasone [13], (2) addition of dimethylsulfoxide (DMSO) [14] and (3) seeding of cells on a collagen matrix [15]. In 1988, Gripon et al. [16] could show that addition of 1.5% DMSO not only preserved hepatocyte function but also markedly enhanced in vitro HBV infection of these cells. Thus, application of DMSO resulting in more frequent and reproducible HBV infections was the basis for further improvements of the in vitro infection model.

After isolation of hepatocytes from liver tissue, cells are seeded onto collagen-coated culture plates. The collagen matrix enhances cell attachment, which is the critical step after cell isolation. Optimal seeding density is crucial, because too high as well as too low cell numbers result in non-confluent monolayers [11] which are no more susceptible for HBV infection in most cases. It has been shown that the loss of intercellular contacts between hepatocytes can lead to impaired hepatocyte function [17], which could explain the negative results of infection experiments using hepatocyte cultures with less than 70% confluence (unpubl. data). Intercellular contacts to non-parenchymal cells can also support hepatocyte function. Typical primary hepatocyte cultures contain 3–15% non-parenchymal cells, which seem to have positive effects on hepatocyte differentiation and susceptibility to in vitro infection [11].

Conditions for in vitro HBV Infection

The major source for infectious viral particles used for in vitro infection experiments are highly viremic serum samples of chronic HBV carriers. But also HBV grown in cultured cells has been shown to successfully infect cultured primary hepatocytes [18, 19]. In this case, viral particles were produced in the human hepatoma cell lines HepG2 or HuH7 after transfection of recombinant replication-competent viral genomic DNA constructs. However, even with culture conditions supporting maintenance of differentiated hepatocytes, in vitro infection efficiency remained rather low. In most experiments, very high virus titers with 100 genome equivalents per hepatocyte or more had to be used for successful infection. In order to improve infection efficiency, Gripon et al. [20] analyzed the effects of polyethylene glycol (PEG) on the infection process. This molecule was chosen because of its fusogenic properties, which may support interaction of the viral envelope and the hepatocyte membrane and consequently enhance viral attachment and penetration. Indeed this study demonstrated that addition of PEG at the time of infection markedly increased infection efficiency. Moreover, the tissue and species specificity of HBV infection was preserved, indicating that the effect of PEG is not a result of unspecific membrane fusion. However, the exact molecular mechanisms of PEG interaction during the infection process are still not defined. The use of HBV particles purified from human serum by gradient centrifugation resulted in increased virus binding and infection efficiency in primary tupaia hepatocyte cultures in the absence of PEG. Addition of HBV-negative human serum inhibited virus binding and infection with these purified virions, indicating the interference of yet unknown serum factors with the infection process [8]. On the other hand, infectious serum samples usually contain large amounts of spherical or filamentous subviral particles, which can be present in a 100- to 100,000-fold excess over infectious virions. During the infection process these non-infectious particles may interfere with the binding of infectious virions, because the filamentous particles carry the pre-S1 domain of the large HBsAg, which is known to mediate viral attachment. With the use of highly purified HBV virions the minimal input virus titer for detectable infection of primary tupaia hepatocytes could be reduced to one genome equivalent per cell without addition of PEG [9]. These data suggest that the PEG-mediated enhancement of infection is restricted to the use of unpurified HBV-containing serum as viral inoculum. One possible explanation for this observation is the previously noted ability of PEG to selectively concentrate HBV virions and as a consequence to support direct interaction between infectious viral particles and target cell membranes [20].

Detection of in vitro HBV Infection

The formation of the covalently closed circular DNA (cccDNA) in primary hepatocyte cultures after HBV inoculation is a reliable marker for successful in vitro infection, because it represents a central step during the viral life cycle and is mediated by cellular polymerases within the nucleus after release of the relaxed circular HBV genome. Southern blot hybridization has been used as standard technique for differentiation between genomic DNA, single-stranded DNA representing a replicative intermediate, and cccDNA [8, 16]. The sensitivity of this method, however, is limited and cccDNA quantity can only roughly be estimated from the signal intensities of hybridized labeled probes. A significantly increased sensitivity of cccDNA detection could be achieved by PCR assays for selective amplification of cccDNA. Finally, application of real-time PCR methods can be used for accurate cccDNA quantification. The amount of cccDNA in infected tupaia hepatocyte cultures has been shown to correlate with input virus titers between 10 and 100 genome equivalents per cell [9, 21].

Immunohistochemical or immunofluorescence staining of infected cells using antibodies directed against the viral surface antigen (HBsAg) or core antigen (HBcAg) is the appropriate method for direct quantification of infection efficiency by determination of the proportion of antigen producing cells. The number of infected cells usually ranges from 5 to 50% depending on infection conditions, different cell preparations, individual viral isolates and quantity of input virus [9, 11, 22]. However, this method gives no information about the transcriptional or replicative activity of individual viral preparations in the specific experimental setting.

Viral transcription can be analyzed by isolation of total mRNA from infected cell cultures and subsequent Northern blot hybridization. Detection of viral transcripts can confirm successful in vitro infection, but sensitivity of Northern blot hybridization is low and assessment of hybridization signal intensities can only differentiate between relative amounts of viral mRNA within the same experiment. Other techniques such as transcriptional analysis by reverse transcription and subsequent PCR amplification (RT-PCR) are more sensitive, but they are not suited for mRNA quantification. However, with the application of real-time PCR technology and the use of specific RNA standards, absolute numbers of viral transcripts can be determined and compared between individual infections. The amount of viral mRNA as measured by real-time PCR has recently been shown to correlate with input virus titers in a range between 1 and 1,000 genome equivalents per hepatocyte, which in turn correlated with the number of infected cells [9, 23].

Detection of cccDNA, immunohistochemical or immunofluorescence staining of intracellular viral antigens and viral RNA quantification are suitable methods for the analysis of in vitro HBV infection. However, these markers only represent the status of viral infection at one defined time point during the course of in vitro infection, because cells have to be lysed for DNA or RNA isolation or fixed for antigen staining. In contrast, detection of viral antigens and DNA in cell culture supernatants can be used for monitoring in vitro viral gene expression and replication. The most accessible markers are HBsAg, hepatitis B virus e antigen (HBeAg) and genomic HBV DNA, which are routinely determined for diagnostic purposes by different immunoassays or PCR systems, respectively. One major difficulty for measuring in vitro antigen and DNA production is the fact that the viral inoculum contains high amounts of HBsAg-containing subviral particles and DNA-containing virus, which are added to the cell culture. After incubation of hepatocytes with the HBV inoculum, subviral particles and unbound virus have to be removed from cell culture by several changes of the culture medium. This can be circumvented by the use of purified virions, as shown by Glebe et al. [9] for in vitro infection of primary tupaia hepatocytes. Removal of subviral particles could significantly reduce input HBsAg and completely eliminate HBeAg from the viral inoculum. De novo synthesis of HBsAg, HBeAg and HBV DNA can then be detected by an increase of viral antigen and DNA during culture of infected hepatocytes [20, 22].

Quantification of Viral Antigen and DNA Production

In most of the former experiments, in vitro production of HBsAg or HBeAg was determined semiquantitatively by commercial radio- or enzyme immunoassays. Relative quantities of viral antigens were assessed by measuring either absolute counts per minute (cpm), signal-to-noise ratio or sample-to-cutoff ratio [20, 22]. These methods are suited for monitoring of viral antigen production during the course of individual infections, but comparison of results from different studies is not possible due to application of different assays and detection protocols. Consequently, the determination of absolute HBsAg concentration (ng/ml) has recently been introduced for the analysis of in vitro HBsAg production [9, 24].

For better characterization of individual infection experiments, quantitative assays not only for HBsAg but also for HBeAg and viral genomic DNA have been introduced. We recently followed the production of HBsAg, HBeAg and HBV DNA quantitatively after infection of primary hepatocytes using real-time PCR for quantification of viral DNA [25]. In these experiments, cells were cultured in 6-well plates on collagen layers. Between days 4 and 6 after plating, infection was performed using highly viremic serum samples in the presence of 5% PEG. Infectivity titers ranged between 50 and 250 genome equivalents per hepatocyte. After an incubation period of 16 h, cell culture supernatants were removed at day 1 post-infection followed by several washing steps at days 2 and 3, and subsequent collection of cell culture supernatants every 24 h for quantitative analysis of HBsAg, HBeAg and viral DNA. Reduction of viral antigens and DNA below levels of de novo synthesis was critical for detection of successful in vitro infection. With the introduction of control experiments using hepatocytes fixed in 70% ethanol prior to the addition of HBV-containing serum, removal of viral antigens and DNA could be followed and directly be compared to the corresponding infection experiment. Results of a representative infection experiment with a standard HBV inoculum are shown in figure 1. After removal of the viral inoculum and washing of the cells, viral antigens and DNA rapidly decreased between days 1 and 3 post-infection. Compared to the negative control, HBsAg reached a steady-state level of in vitro production on day 6 post-infection at a concentration of approximately 100 ng/ml per 24 h whereas HBeAg markedly increased on day 4 to a peak antigen concentration of 10 ng/ml on day 8. Levels of HBV DNA decreased from 4.0×10^8 copies/ml of viral input to 2.0×10^5 copies/ml during washing steps and reached a concentration of 1.6×10^6 copies/ml at the maximum of HBV replication.

Standardization of in vitro HBV Infection

Inter-experimental variability of HBsAg production measured by a commercial radioimmunoassay has been reported to be considerably high with values between 1,000 and 15,000 cpm per 24 h corresponding to relative HBsAg amounts differing about a factor of 15 [22]. The variations between these different experiments are mainly due to the high variability of different preparations of human hepatocytes. This is most probably the major cause for the limited reproducibility of experiments using different donor cells. Because total amounts of human hepatocytes from single cell preparations are usually limited and infection experiments are very laborious, the number of different experiments which can be performed with cells from the same hepatocyte preparation is in most cases restricted to a maximum of 20–30. Thus, for a major improvement of the human infection model, standardized infection and

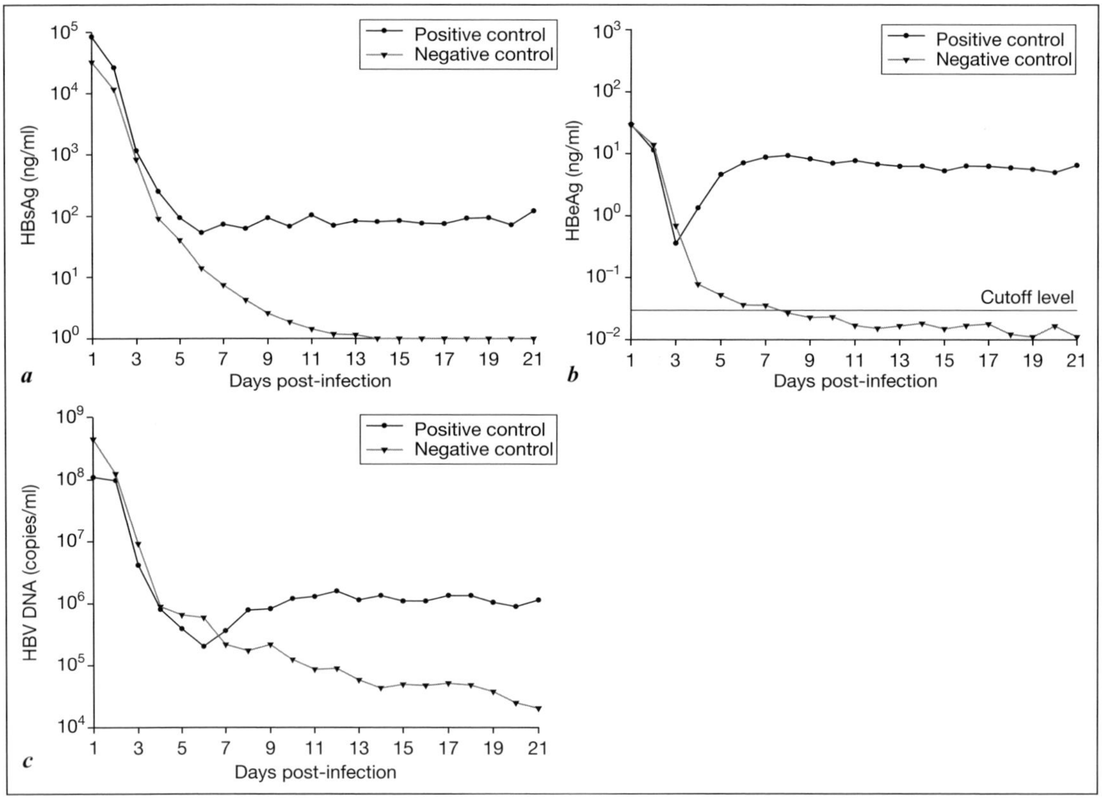

Fig. 1. Time course of in vitro production of HBsAg (***a***), HBeAg (***b***) and HBV DNA (***c***) after infection of primary human hepatocytes with a standard HBV inoculum. For negative controls, cells were fixed in 70% ethanol prior to addition of the HBV inoculum.

evaluation procedures should be introduced, which would at least to a certain extent allow a direct comparison of results from infection experiments with cells from different donors.

Assessment of susceptibility of hepatocytes from different donors is crucial for direct comparison of inter-experimental results. Application of constant culture and infection conditions and quantification of in vitro production of HBsAg, HBeAg and viral DNA provide the basis for standardization of experiments with different hepatocyte cultures. The maximum concentrations of HBsAg, HBeAg and HBV DNA measured during the culture period after in vitro infection seem to be useful parameters for characterization of infection experiments with hepatocytes from individual donors, because these values are independent of variable kinetics of in vitro antigen and DNA synthesis. The maximum production of

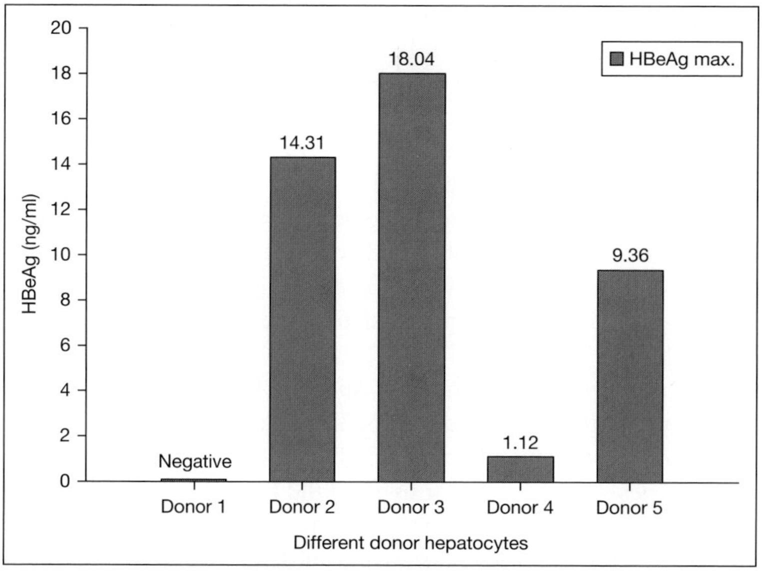

Fig. 2. Maximum in vitro HBeAg production after infection of primary human hepatocytes from 5 different donors with a standard HBV inoculum.

viral antigens and DNA following infection with a standard HBV inoculum could be used as a measure for the infectibility of a particular hepatocyte preparation. In a series of experiments using five different hepatocyte preparations, we analyzed maximum HBeAg production after infection with a standard HBV inoculum. Maximum HBeAg levels varied from 0 to 18.0 ng/ml (fig. 2) reflecting the high variation of infectibility of different cell preparations. Thus, production of viral antigens and DNA seems to depend to a great extent on the hepatocyte preparation used and will considerably differ between experiments with cells from different donors. The application of a standard control infection therefore seems to be essential to characterize the infectibility of a particular donor cell preparation. Maximum values of viral antigen and DNA production obtained with the positive control for each HBV inoculum can then serve as points of reference for infections under different experimental conditions.

Applications for the Human in vitro Infection Model

Viral Attachment and Cellular Receptor Studies

An important application for the human in vitro infection model is the analysis of the molecular interactions between HBV and target cells during the early steps of viral replication. Several investigations based on infection of primary human hepatocytes have already confirmed results obtained from binding studies with non-permissive hepatoma cell lines [26]. With these experiments different epitopes within the pre-S1 domain of the large HBsAg could be identified, which are involved in viral attachment. It has been shown that binding of specific antibodies within the N-terminal region of the pre-S1 domain harboring the attachment site can completely block in vitro infection [27–30]. However, the respective host cell receptor mediating pre-S1-dependent binding of HBV and putative co-receptors have not been identified so far, although several cellular proteins have been proposed as possible candidates [31–33].

Determination of Neutralizing Activity of Specific Antibodies

Besides the neutralizing activity of antibodies against the pre-S1 region, protective immunity is predominantly mediated by antibodies directed towards conformational epitopes within the major hydrophilic loop (MHL) of the small HBsAg. Amino acid exchanges within the MHL may lead to alterations of the three-dimensional structure of these epitopes and subsequently to reduced antibody binding [34]. Emergence of viral variants with mutations within the MHL can cause recurrent HBV infection after liver transplantation in spite of passive immunization with polyclonal human hepatitis B immunoglobulin [35]. This observation has led to the assumption that there is a direct correlation between reduced antibody binding and loss of neutralizing activity. In order to prove this hypothesis, an in vitro neutralization assay based on primary human hepatocytes has been established. Analysis of the neutralizing activity of monoclonal and polyclonal antibodies against HBsAg has been done by preincubation of the viral inoculum with the respective antibodies and subsequent in vitro infection. With this method, Ryu et al. [36] have demonstrated that monoclonal antibodies against a conformational epitope within the MHL of HBsAg could block in vitro infection completely. These monoclonal antibodies had an approximately 2,000 times higher inhibitory activity than polyclonal human hepatitis B immunoglobulin.

Analysis of Antiviral Effects of Cytokines

During acute and chronic HBV infection, different antiviral cytokines are produced by cells of the innate and adaptive immune system. Specifically, interferon-γ (IFN-γ) and tumor necrosis factor-α (TNF-α) have been shown to play an important role for viral clearance and immunopathogenesis of HBV infection. Both cytokines can inhibit viral replication in HBV transgenic mice expressing single viral antigens or complete viral genomes without destroying antigen- or virus-producing hepatocytes [37, 38]. In order to characterize the antiviral effect of IFN-γ on HBV-infected hepatocytes, Lau et al. [39] and Suri

15 Rojkind M, Gatmaitan Z, Mackensen S, Giambrone MA, Ponce P, Reid LM: Connective tissue biomatrix: Its isolation and utilization for long-term cultures of normal rat hepatocytes. J Cell Biol 1980;87:255–263.
16 Gripon P, Diot C, Thézé N, Fourel I, Loreal O, Brechot C, Guguen-Guillouzo C: Hepatitis B virus infection of adult human hepatocytes cultured in the presence of dimethylsulfoxide. J Virol 1988;62:4136–4143.
17 Hamilton GA, Jolley SL, Gilbert D, Coon DJ, Barros S, LeCluyse EL: Regulation of cell morphology and cytochrome P_{450} expression in human hepatocytes by extracellular matrix and cell-cell interactions. Cell Tissue Res 2001;306:85–99.
18 Gripon P, Le Seyec J, Rumin S, Guguen-Guillouzo C: Myristylation of the hepatitis B virus large surface protein is essential for viral infectivity. Virology 1995;213:292–299.
19 Protzer U, Nassal M, Chiang PW, Kirschfink M, Schaller H: Interferon gene transfer by a hepatitis B virus vector efficiently suppresses wild-type virus infection. Proc Natl Acad Sci USA 1999;96:10818–10823.
20 Gripon P, Diot C, Guguen-Guillouzo C: Reproducible high level infection of cultured adult human hepatocytes by hepatitis B virus: Effect of polyethylene glycol on adsorption and penetration. Virology 1993;192:534–540.
21 He ML, Wu J, Chen Y, Lin MC, Lau GK, Kung HF: A new and sensitive method for the quantification of HBV cccDNA by real-time PCR. Biochem Biophys Res Commun 2002;295:1102–1107.
22 Galle PR, Hagelstein J, Kommerell B, Volkmann M, Schranz P, Zentgraf H: In vitro experimental infection of primary human hepatocytes with hepatitis B virus. Gastroenterology 1994;106: 664–673.
23 Jursch CA, Gerlich WH, Glebe D, Schaefer S, Marie O, Thraenhart O: Molecular approaches to validate disinfectants against human hepatitis B virus. Med Microbiol Immunol 2002;190:189–197.
24 Ren S, Nassal M: Hepatitis B virus (HBV) virion and covalently closed circular DNA formation in primary tupaia hepatocytes and human hepatoma cell lines upon HBV genome transduction with replication-defective adenovirus vectors. J Virol 2001;75:1104–1116.
25 Weinberger KM, Wiedenmann E, Böhm S, Jilg W: Sensitive and accurate quantitation of hepatitis B virus DNA using a kinetic fluorescence detection system (TaqMan PCR). J Virol Methods 2000;85:75–82.
26 De Meyer S, Gong ZJ, Suwandhi W, van Pelt J, Soumillion A, Yap SH: Organ and species specificity of hepatitis B virus (HBV) infection: A review of literature with special reference to preferential attachment of HBV to human hepatocytes. J Viral Hepat 1997;4:145–153.
27 Le Seyec J, Chouteau P, Cannie I, Guguen-Guillouzo C, Gripon P: Role of the pre-S2 domain of the large envelope protein in hepatitis B virus assembly and infectivity. J Virol 1998;72:5573–5578.
28 Le Seyec J, Chouteau P, Cannie I, Guguen-Guillouzo C, Gripon P: Infection process of the hepatitis B virus depends on the presence of a defined sequence in the pre-S1 domain. J Virol 1999;73:2052–2057.
29 Maeng CY, Ryu CJ, Gripon P, Guguen-Guillouzo C, Hong HJ: Fine mapping of virus-neutralizing epitopes on hepatitis B virus pre-S1. Virology 2000;270:9–16.
30 Chouteau P, Le Seyec J, Cannie I, Nassal M, Guguen-Guillouzo C, Gripon P: A short N-proximal region of the large envelope protein harbors a determinant that contributes to the species specificity of human hepatitis B virus. J Virol 2001;75:11565–11572.
31 Mabit H, Vons C, Dubanchet S, Capel F, Franco D, Petit MA: Primary cultured normal human hepatocytes for hepatitis B virus receptor studies. J Hepatol 1996;24:403–412.
32 Treichel U, Meyer zum Büschenfelde KH, Dienes HP, Gerken G: Receptor-mediated entry of hepatitis B virus particles into liver cells. Arch Virol 1997;142:493–498.
33 Paran N, Cooper A, Shaul Y: Interaction of hepatitis B virus with cells. Rev Med Virol 2003;13: 137–143.
34 Zuckerman AJ: Effect of hepatitis B virus mutants on efficacy of vaccination. Lancet 2000;355: 1382–1384.
35 Protzer-Knolle U, Naumann U, Bartenschlager R, Berg T, Hopf U, Meyer zum Büschenfelde KH, Neuhaus P, Gerken G: Hepatitis B virus with antigenically altered hepatitis B surface antigen is selected by high-dose hepatitis B immune globulin after liver transplantation. Hepatology 1998;27:254–263.

36 Ryu CJ, Gripon P, Park HR, Park SS, Kim YK, Guguen-Guillouzo C, Yoo OJ, Hong HJ: In vitro neutralization of hepatitis B virus by monoclonal antibodies against the viral surface antigen. J Med Virol 1997;52:226–233.
37 Guidotti LG, Ishikawa T, Hobbs MV, Matzke B, Schreiber R, Chisari FV: Intracellular inactivation of the hepatitis B virus by cytotoxic T lymphocytes. Immunity 1996;4:25–36.
38 McClary H, Koch R, Chisari FV, Guidotti LG: Relative sensitivity of hepatitis B virus and other hepatotropic viruses to the antiviral effects of cytokines. J Virol 2000;74:2255–2264.
39 Lau JYN, Bain VG, Naoumov NV, Smith HM, Alexander GJM, Williams R: Effect of interferon-γ on hepatitis B viral antigen expression in primary hepatocyte culture. Hepatology 1991;14: 975–979.
40 Suri D, Schilling R, Lopes AR, Mullerova I, Colucci G, Williams R, Naoumov NV: Non-cytolytic inhibition of hepatitis B virus replication in human hepatocytes. J Hepatol 2001;35:790–797.
41 Rehermann B: Immune responses in hepatitis B virus infection. Semin Liver Dis 2003;23:21–37.
42 Ando K, Guidotti LG, Wirth S, Ishikawa T, Missale G, Moriyama T, Schreiber RD, Schlicht HJ, Huang S, Chisari FV: Class I-restricted cytotoxic T lymphocytes are directly cytopathic for their target cells in vivo. J Immunol 1994;152:3245–3253.
43 Franco A, Guidotti LG, Hobbs MV, Pasquetto V, Chisari FV: Pathogenetic effector function of CD4-positive T-helper 1 cells in hepatitis B virus transgenic mice. J Immunol 1997;159: 2001–2008.
44 Zoulim F: Assessing hepatitis B virus resistance in vitro and molecular mechanisms of nucleoside resistance. Semin Liver Dis 2002;22(suppl 1):23–31.
45 De Clercq E: Perspectives for the treatment of hepatitis B virus infections. Int J Antimicrob Agents 1999;12:81–95.
46 Gripon P, Rumin S, Urban S, Le Seyec J, Glaise D, Cannie I, Guyomard C, Lucas J, Trepo C, Guguen-Guillouzo C: Infection of a human hepatoma cell line by hepatitis B virus. Proc Natl Acad Sci USA 2002;99:15655–15660.
47 Köck J, Baumert TF, Delaney WE, Blum HE, von Weizsäcker F: Inhibitory effect of adefovir and lamivudine on the initiation of hepatitis B virus infection in primary tupaia hepatocytes. Hepatology 2003;38:1410–1418.

Stephan Boehm
Institute for Medical Microbiology and Hygiene, University of Regensburg
Franz-Josef-Strauss-Allee 11, DE–93053 Regensburg (Germany)
Tel. +49 941 9446490, Fax +49 941 9446402
E-Mail stephan.boehm@klinik.uni-regensburg.de

von Weizsäcker F, Roggendorf M (eds): Models of Viral Hepatitis.
Monogr Virol. Basel, Karger, 2005, vol 25, pp 135–145

Progress and Perspectives of the uPA/RAG-2 Mouse Model: Liver Repopulation and Viral Infection Studies

Maura Dandri, Martin R. Burda, Urte Matschl, Karsten Wursthorn, Joerg Petersen

Department of Medicine, University Hospital Hamburg-Eppendorf, and Heinrich-Pette-Institute for Experimental Virology and Immunology, University of Hamburg, Hamburg, Germany

Hepatocyte Transplantation

Liver transplantation is a successful and well-established treatment for end-stage liver disease and liver failure. However, donor organ scarcity is a fundamental limitation of this therapy. The availability of highly differentiated primary liver cells to be used for cell-based therapies, such as hepatocyte transplantation, tissue-engineered organs, or for extracorporeal liver support systems represents an attractive alternative to whole organ transplantation [1, 2]. Freshly isolated normal adult hepatocytes are already widely used in various research areas of hepatology, pharmacology and toxicology, and initial clinical trials have also shown their potential for therapeutic applications [3]. Essential prerequisites for therapeutic use of hepatocyte transplantation in people is that primary liver cells must be promptly available, remain highly differentiated and maintain their proliferative capabilities within the host liver, since only a limited number of cells can be infused into a patient [4]. Although techniques for the isolation of hepatocytes from human livers are continuing to improve, primary human hepatocytes are difficult to maintain in culture in a differentiated state. The cells lose their capacity to secrete liver-specific enzymes such as albumin or α_1-antitrypsin and they become non-permissive for hepatotropic viruses, such as hepatitis B virus (HBV) and hepatitis C virus (HCV), very fast after plating. Therefore, any system which will allow to maintain hepatocytes in a highly differentiated status and, eventually, cell growth, will offer unique opportunities to address studies on hepatocyte biology and hepatotropic viruses for which no cell lines or convenient animal models exist.

The uPA/RAG-2 Mouse Model

Liver repopulation with hepatocyte transplantation has significant potential for gene therapy applications and analysis of fundamental biological mechanisms in metabolic and viral diseases [2–3, 5]. Various models have been developed in recent years utilizing human liver tissues or isolated primary hepatocytes for transplantation into immunocompromised mice [6–10]. Those studies documented that transplanted hepatocytes can integrate into the host liver parenchyma, though engrafted cells showed very limited proliferative activity in the normal liver. Studies in transgenic mice have shown that the liver can be repopulated by genetically engineered rodent hepatocytes harboring a selective growth advantage over resident hepatocytes [11–15]. The discovery of a liver-toxic phenotype in urokinase-type plasminogen activator (uPA) transgenic mice led to the development of a novel liver repopulation model, in which hepatocyte-targeted overexpression of the albumin-uPA transgene leads to the death of transgene-carrying hepatocytes, resulting in a growth advantage for transplanted cells. Cell damage appears to be due to intracellular activation of the uPA substrate plasminogen, which in turn would activate plasmin and induce proteolytic damage within the rough endoplasmic reticulum. However, transgene deletion takes place in some endogenous mouse hepatocytes and those cells are competitively growing with transplanted hepatocytes [12, 13]. In this mouse model, hepatocyte proliferative stimulus lasts approximately 8 weeks after birth, until the transplanted hepatocyte mass becomes comparable to the hepatocyte mass in the liver of non-transgenic normal mice [7, 13, 16]. To address studies on human liver diseases and hepatotropic viruses, for which no permissive cell lines exist, we bred hemizygous alb-uPA mice with immunocompromised RAG-2 knock-out mice. The RAG-2 mice lack mature T and B lymphocytes due to a deletion in the recombination activation gene 2 (RAG-2) [17].

Transplantation of Adult Human Primary Hepatocytes

Within the last years, the feasibility of human hepatocyte transplantation in the liver of immunodeficient uPA transgenic mice was demonstrated [7, 10]. We transplant uPA/RAG-2 mice with adult primary human hepatocytes isolated from the normal adult liver [7]. Using standard collagenase perfusion techniques, we isolate primary human hepatocytes from donor liver specimens that are not utilized for human liver transplantation, and from surgical liver tissues remaining after partial hepatectomy. Hepatocytes are transplanted into 2- to 3-week-old uPA/RAG-2 mice by intrasplenic injection. To screen for survival and engraftment of transplanted human hepatocytes, serum albumin profiles are analyzed by immunoblotting using a specific monoclonal antibody that does not cross-react with any mouse serum protein. Human albumin is specifically found in uPA/RAG-2 mice sera containing human hepatocytes [7]. To evaluate the ratio of human versus mouse serum albumin in transplanted mice, test mixtures of human and mouse sera are analyzed in parallel and signal intensities on the blots are quantified by densitometry. Levels of human albumin usually range between 0.5 and 15% in the sera of successfully transplanted mice, strongly indicating that transplanted human hepatocytes engrafted and survived in the uPA/RAG-2 livers. To directly demonstrate human hepatocyte engraftment into the liver of uPA/RAG-2 mice, livers are screened for the presence of human-specific genome sequences by PCR. Genomic DNA extracted both from human and mouse liver specimens are amplified by PCR using primers specific for a fraction of highly repeated human *Alu* sequences. A single band of the expected size is exclusively amplified when DNAs extracted either from human or uPA/RAG-2 mouse livers successfully transplanted with human hepatocytes are used [7]. We did not detect human DNA in tissues other than the liver. This observation is in agreement with previous reports showing that intrasplenic injection of normal hepatocytes in mice does not favor persisting cell engraftment in tissues other than the liver [4, 16]. uPA/RAG-2 mice containing human hepatocytes are clinically healthy and the livers appear normal in respect to color, size and liver to body weight ratios at sacrifice. Approximately 80% of transplanted mice survived the procedure. The most common reason for death of transplanted young mice was a diffuse bleeding complication due to the overexpression of uroplasminogen. By screening of the mice for the production of human serum albumin, we estimated that engraftment of human hepatocytes was successful in approximately 70% of the transplanted mice, when mice were transplanted with highly viable hepatocytes (≥80%). Viable hepatocytes could be isolated from partially hepatectomized livers that underwent a considerable time of warm ischemia before perfusion (2–4 h), but cell viability was lower (40–80%) and transplantation into mice was not successful. Hepatocytes that had been liberated from cirrhotic livers or from healthy donors in other liver centers, and were sent to us as cell solutions, were also not successfully transplanted.

HBV Infection of Transplanted Hepatocytes in Mice

HBV infection is a major public health problem and an important cause of infectious disease mortality worldwide. Approximately 2 billion people have serologic evidence of past or present HBV infection, and 350 million people are chronically infected. Each year over 1 million people die from HBV-related chronic liver disease, including cirrhosis and hepatocellular carcinoma [18]. Unfortunately, the efficiency of current therapeutic strategies such as interferon-α or inhibitors of HBV DNA polymerase (adefovir dipivoxil, lamivudine) is limited [19–21] and the effectiveness of innovative therapeutic approaches, such as inhibitors of HBV core capsid formation, still remains to be evaluated in vivo [22]. The understanding of the complete viral life cycle, as well as the development of more effective antiviral drugs aiming at the complete eradication of the virus from chronic carriers, have been hampered by the lack of efficient in vitro infection systems and suitable animal models. Therefore, to test whether transplanted human hepatocytes were useful for HBV studies, uPA/RAG-2 mice were injected with HBV infectious human serum. Serum samples were collected between 2 weeks and 2 months after inoculation and analyzed for the presence of surface antigen (HBsAg) by ELISA and HBV DNA by real-time PCR. HBV-injected mice became HBsAg positive approximately 8 weeks after inoculation [7, and unpubl. data]. High levels of HBV DNA (1×10^7 to 1×10^8 genome equivalents/ml serum) were found in sera of uPA/RAG-2 mice transplanted with human hepatocytes, whereas no viral DNA was detectable in no transplanted but HBV-injected mice. The absence of HBV-DNA in no transplanted mice demonstrates that positive signals could not have resulted from the original injection and, as expected, that mice not containing human hepatocytes are not susceptible to hepatitis B virus infection. The expression of HBV-specific genes represents an unequivocal marker to distinguish between mouse host and transplanted human hepatocytes and permits a rough estimation of the number of successfully transplanted and functional hepatocytes in mouse livers. Therefore, mouse liver sections randomly chosen from different lobes were immunohistochemically stained for hepatitis B core antigen (HBcAg). HBcAg-positive hepatocytes were found as clusters throughout the uPA/RAG-2 mouse livers and, as expected [16], grouped around portal veins and in adjacent areas [7]. Inspection of multiple cryostat sections for each of the transplanted and infected mice revealed HBcAg-positive staining, whereas none were positive in non-transplanted but HBV-injected mice. Histological examination of various extrahepatic tissues of transplanted mice, such as spleen, lungs and peritoneum, was in line with our DNA data and failed to identify surviving hepatocytes in those organs [7].

Previous studies indicated that only approximately 20% of splenically injected cells reach the liver and survive (that corresponds in our experiments to about 1 × 10^5 cells), while a mouse liver contains about 1 × 10^8 hepatocytes [23]. In this case, engraftment without repopulation could result in only 0.1–0.5% human hepatocytes in transplanted mice. The presence of 0.5–15% human hepatocytes in several mouse livers, as indicated by the levels of human albumin in the serum, human genomic DNA in the liver, as well as by the number of HBcAg-positive hepatocytes, strongly suggests that each transplanted human hepatocyte may have undergone several cell doublings, provided all transplanted cells proliferated equally. Based on these data and considerations, human hepatocytes have shown to maintain the capability to proliferate to a certain extent in the uPA/RAG-2 mouse liver.

Hepadnaviral Infection of Mice Repopulated with Tupaia Hepatocytes

We showed that human hepatocytes transplanted in uPA/RAG-2 mice are suitable for studies on HBV infection [7]. However, the availability of viable human hepatocytes is a major limitation of these studies. Therefore, we recently explored the potential use of primary hepatocytes isolated from *Tupaia belangeri*, a squirrel-like animal phylogenetically related to primates [24], to establish a new infection model in immunosuppressed uPA/RAG-2 mice. Primary tupaia hepatocytes (PTH) were previously found to be reproducibly susceptible to infection with HBV and woolly monkey hepatitis B virus (WM-HBV) in vitro [25–28], while infection of tree shrews themselves is transient and the level of gene expression and viral replication in the liver of these animals are rather low [25].

To determine the extent of engraftment of tupaia hepatocytes, transplanted uPA/RAG-2 mice were screened for the production of tupaia α_1-antitrypsin (TAAT). TAAT profiles were analyzed by immunoblotting using a monoclonal antibody that allows the specific identification of human and tupaia AAT in mouse serum. We estimated that hepatocyte engraftment was successful (TAAT $\geq$10%) in approximately 80% of the transplanted mice [29]. Furthermore, long-term repopulation studies showed that the production of TAAT remained stable in all mice during the entire observation time of up to 1 year. Sections from transplanted livers showed large nodules of tupaia hepatocytes arranged in typical cord-like structures. Within xenogenic nodules, hepatocyte cytoplasm and nuclei appeared histologically normal compared with the surrounding mouse liver. The extent of mouse liver repopulation ranged between 30 and 80%, and correlated with the TAAT titers in serum [manuscript submitted].

Our studies showed that highly differentiated PTH are able to engraft xenogenic mouse livers with high efficiency. Using the previously described hemizygous uPA/RAG-2 mice [7, 16] it was possible to achieve repopulation levels (up to 80%) comparable to the values found after transplantation of woodchuck hepatocytes [16] or other rodent hepatocytes [13, 22, 30]. This is substantially higher than the repopulation levels achieved with adult human hepatocytes [7]. One of the reasons for the different efficacies may be the ex situ isolation method used for human hepatocytes, where the tissues are first flushed with a preserving solution and then perfused in vitro. On the other hand, the liver of laboratory animals is perfused in situ without intermediate steps which may have a negative impact on engraftment or expansion capacity of the transplanted hepatocytes, though the viability both for human and tupaia cells was similar. It is also possible that cross-talk with non-parenchymal cells, matrix and growth factors in mice is more efficient for PTH compared to human hepatocytes. It is known that hepatocytes transplantation into hemizygous uPA/RAG-2 mice results in a competition between transplanted and endogenously recombined mouse hepatocytes in the diseased mouse liver tissue [13, 16]. Tupaia hepatocytes having a growth advantage compared to human hepatocytes in the mouse liver would therefore repopulate the mouse liver with greater efficiency.

Our experiments show that hemizygous uPA/RAG-2 mice repopulated with tupaia hepatocytes can be infected with HBV-positive human serum [manuscript submitted, 29]. Successfully infected mice developed prolonged HBV infection associated with high viral titers. Both human HBV and WM-HBV can infect uPA/RAG-2 mice transplanted with tupaia hepatocytes, confirming the results from in vitro cultivated PTH [26]. WM-HBsAg was already detectable at 6 weeks post-inoculation, whereas HBV-HBsAg started showing positive reactions in the ELISA at 12 weeks post-inoculation. The longer lag time for productive HBV infection may be due to the fact that the evolutionary differences between the natural host of WM-HBV, the woolly monkey, and tupaia are smaller than between tupaia and humans [31]. Therefore, virus/host interactions between WM-HBV and PTH may be more efficient than the interactions of human HBV with tupaia cells. This is in accordance with the in vitro data obtained by Köck et al. [26], who observed a lower replication rate of HBV compared to WM-HBV in plated PTH. We performed serum passage experiments to establish that PTH support the full replication cycle of HBV and WM-HBV. Furthermore, sequence analysis failed to reveal the emergence of new viral populations in HBV-infected mice, both before and after passage experiments, indicating that a strong selective pressure is not required to establish HBV infection in TPH repopulated mice [29, manuscript submitted].

As shown recently in humans with chronic HBV infection, total intracellular and cccDNA in hepatocytes can be accurately quantified using real-time PCR [32]. We applied this method to tupaia repopulated mice infected with WM-HBV and HBV. Quantification with real-time PCR revealed the presence of cccDNA, approximately 25–100 cccDNA copies per tupaia liver cell, in WM-HBV-infected tupaia-chimeric mice, while the intracellular titers of total

WM-HBV DNA ranged between 3 and 12 × 10^3 copies per cell, respectively [manuscript submitted]. Total intracellular and cccDNA amounts were also analyzed in liver tissues obtained from 1 HBV-positive mouse that had been sacrificed 6 months after infection. The levels of cccDNA (35 molecules per tupaia cell) and intracellular total viral DNA (3.8 × 10^3) were in the same range as in WM-HBV-infected mice [manuscript submitted]. Interestingly, the ratio of intracellular total DNA vs. cccDNA in grafted mice was within the range found in HBV chronically infected human livers [32]. Detection and determination of cccDNA amounts in infected mice indicate that this chimeric mouse model is suitable for studying cccDNA amplification and cccDNA half-life in vivo. Together, our infection experiments show that in the chimeric tupaia/uPA/RAG-2 mice the viral cycle is complete and infectious viral particles are produced for the life span of the animals.

One of the major applications of a hepatitis B mouse model is the ability to test antiviral substances. To demonstrate the usefulness of the chimeric tupaia/mouse system for antiviral studies, 2 adult chimeric mice with persistently high levels of WM-HBV were treated with adefovir dipivoxil [manuscript submitted]. The viral titers dropped in both mice of 2 logs after 10 weeks of treatment, and returned to the original values within 3 weeks of drug withdrawal, thus demonstrating the specific antiviral effect of adefovir dipivoxil on WM-HBV. Altogether, the prompt responsiveness to antiviral drug treatment indicates that uPA/RAG-2 mice repopulated with TPH are suitable for long-term antiviral studies, which is a major limitation of the antiviral drug evaluation performed in vitro using primary hepatocyte cultures.

Cryopreservation and Transplantation of Frozen Primary Hepatocytes

Due to the scarce availability of fresh human livers, cryopreservation and effective recovery of primary human hepatocytes are highly needed for various therapeutic applications. Experiments with rat hepatocytes have demonstrated that thawed cells retain various functions, such as drug-metabolizing enzyme activities, when cultured under specific conditions [33]. These findings indicate that cryopreserved hepatocytes may retain their regenerative capacity after thawing, which is a fundamental requirement for potential therapeutic applications in the future. We presented a protocol which allowed cryopreservation and efficient recovery of primary hepatocytes isolated from adult woodchucks [34]. We showed that cryopreserved primary woodchuck hepatocytes retained their proliferative potential in vivo, when transplanted into immunodeficient uPA/RAG-2 mice [34]. Our in vivo infection studies also indicated that susceptibility for infection with WHV in mice harboring cryopreserved cells was comparable to that observed by infecting animals containing fresh woodchuck hepatocytes.

Efficient repopulation of uPA/RAG-2 mouse livers and establishment of hepadnavirus infection was also achieved with cryopreserved PTH [manuscript submitted]. We estimated that hepatocyte engraftment was successful (TAAT $\geq$10%) in approximately 80 and 70% of the mice transplanted with fresh or cryopreserved PTH, respectively. Due to the limited window available for transplantation in the uPA/RAG-2 mice, the ability to use cryopreserved tupaia liver cells offers the opportunity to perform transplantation experiments at any time.

Recently, several transplantation experiments have been performed by our group using also cryopreserved human liver cells. The use of our freeze-thaw protocol permitted long term preservation (longer than 1 year) and successful transplantation of hepatocytes isolated from humans [unpubl. data]. Results based both on histological evaluation and on measurement of human albumin levels in mouse sera revealed that transplantation efficiency was still high (approx. 50%) when cryopreserved cells were used, though slightly lower repopulation levels (up to 5%) were achieved in successfully transplanted mice.

Further Applications

The ability to establish productive HBV infection in mice transplanted with human or tupaia hepatocytes indicates that such a system will allow analysis of viral biology in a convenient small animal model. uPA/RAG-2 mice harboring human or tupaia primary hepatocytes have been shown to allow studies of the full HBV viral replication cycle. This will be of particular value for in vivo testing of novel antiviral compounds and other therapeutic drugs using rather small amounts of compounds. From our experience, it appears that the most critical and limiting factor to succeed in transplantation of normal human hepatocytes in these mice is the scarce availability of healthy liver tissues that underwent a very short ischemia time before perfusion. However, the knowledge that human hepatocytes can engraft and partially repopulate a xenogenic liver opens new exciting possibilities to develop novel experimental models for studies on other hepatotropic viruses. The report of Mercer et al. [10] showed that transplantation of normal human hepatocytes into homozygous immunodeficient uPA mice led to repopulation of diseased mouse livers with transplanted cells that were susceptible to chronic HCV infection. However, productive HCV infection was not achieved when hemizygous uPA mice were used [10, and pers. unpubl data]. Establishment of a homozygous uPA colony appears to be very difficult, both due to the high mortality of these animals in utero and within the first 2 weeks after birth and due to the low fertility of the homozygous mice [pers. observations]. Therefore, further transplantation experiments in hemizygous mice using alternative sources of cells, such as tupaia liver cells that were shown to be susceptible to HCV infection in vitro [35], are under investigation in order to determine the capability of these cells to sustain HCV infection in the mouse liver environment.

Moreover, the uPA mouse model provides new tools to characterize the biology of human hepatocytes, as well as to explore the potential of bone marrow-derived and peripheral liver progenitor cells in the process of liver regeneration.

Acknowledgments

This work was supported by a grant from the Deutsche Forschungsgemeinschaft to J.P. (Pe608/2-3) and from the German Hepatitis network Hep-Net.

References

1 Gupta S, Rajvanshi P, Bhargava Kerr A: Hepatocyte transplantation: Progress toward liver repopulation. Prog Liver Dis 1996;14:199–222.
2 Lake JR: Hepatocyte transplantation. N Engl J Med 1998;338:1463–1465.
3 Fox IJ, Chowdhury JR, Kaufman SS, Goertzen TC, Chowdhury NR, Warkentin PI, Dorko K, et al: Treatment of the Crigler-Najjar syndrome type I with hepatocyte transplantation. N Engl J Med 1998;338:1422–1426.
4 Gupta S, Bhargava KK, Novikoff PM: Mechanisms of cell engraftment during liver repopulation with hepatocyte transplantation. Semin Liver Dis 1999;19:15–26.
5 Vemuru RP, Aragona E, Gupta S: Analysis of hepatocellular proliferation: Study of archival liver tissue is facilitated by an endogenous marker of DNA replication. Hepatology 1992;16:968–973.
6 Brown JJ, Parashar B, Moshage H, et al: A long-term hepatitis B viremia model generated by transplanting nontumorigenic immortalized human hepatocytes in Rag-2-deficient mice. Hepatology 2000;31:173–181.
7 Dandri M, Burda MR, Iwanska A, Sommer G, Török E, Pollok JM, Rogiers X, Gupta S, Will H, Greten H, Petersen J: Repopulation of mouse liver with human hepatocytes and in vivo infection with hepatitis B virus. Hepatology 2001;33:981–988.
8 Ilan E, Burakova T, Dagan S, Nussbaum O, Lubin I, Eren R, Ben-Moshe O, et al: The hepatitis B virus-trimera mouse: A model for human HBV infection and evaluation of anti-HBV therapeutic agents. Hepatology 1999;29:553–562.
9 Ohashi K, Marion PL, Nakai H, Meuse L, Cullen JM, Bordier BB, Schwall R, et al: Sustained survival of human hepatocytes in mice: A model for in vivo infection with human hepatitis B and hepatitis delta viruses. Nat Med 2000;6:327–331.
10 Mercer DF, Schiller DE, Elliott JF, Douglas DN, Hao C, Rinfret A, Addison WR, et al: Hepatitis C virus replication in mice with chimeric human livers. Nat Med 2001;7:927–933.
11 Gupta S, Rajvanshi P, Aragona E, Lee CD, Yerneni PR, Burk RD: Transplanted hepatocytes proliferate differently after CCl4 treatment and hepatocyte growth factor infusion. Am J Physiol 1999;276:G629–G638.

12 Sandgren EP, Palmiter RD, Heckel JL, Daugherty CC, Brinster RL, Degen JL: Complete hepatic regeneration after somatic deletion of an albumin-plasminogen activator transgene. Cell 1991;66: 245–256.

13 Rhim JA, Sandgren EP, Degen JL, Palmiter RD, Brinster RL: Replacement of diseased mouse liver by hepatic cell transplantation. Science 1994;263:1149–1152.

14 Overturf K, Al-Dhalimy M, Tanguay R, et al: Hepatocytes corrected by gene therapy are selected in vivo in a murine model of hereditary tyrosinaemia type I. Nat Genet 1996;12:266–273. Erratum in: Nat Genet 1996;12:458.

15 Mignon A, Guidotti JE, Mitchell C, et al: Selective repopulation of normal mouse liver by Fas/CD95-resistant hepatocytes. Nat Med 1998;4:1185–1188.

16 Petersen J, Dandri M, Gupta S, Rogler CE: Liver repopulation with xenogenic hepatocytes in B-and T-cell-deficient mice leads to chronic hepadnavirus infection and clonal growth of hepatocellular carcinoma. Proc Natl Acad Sci USA 1998;95:310–315.

17 Shinkai Y, Rathbun G, Lam KP, et al: RAG-2-deficient mice lack mature lymphocytes owing to inability to initiate V(D)J rearrangement. Cell 1992;68:855–867.

18 Alter MJ: Epidemiology and prevention of hepatitis B. Semin Liver Dis 2003;23:3946.

19 Marcellin P, Chang TT, Lim SG, Tong MJ, Sievert W, Shiffmann ML, Jeffers L, et al: Adefovir dipivoxil for the treatment of hepatitis Be antigen-positive chronic hepatitis B. N Engl J Med 2003;348:808–816.

20 Hadziyannis SJ, Tassopoulos NC, Heathcote EJ, Chang TT, Kitis G, Rizzetto M, Marcellin P, et al: Adefovir dipivoxil for the treatment of hepatitis Be antigen-negative chronic hepatitis B. N Engl J Med 2003;348:800–807.

21 Chin R, Locarnini S: Treatment of chronic hepatitis B: Current challenges and future directions. Rev Med Virol 2003;13:255–272.

22 Deres K, Schroder CH, Paessens A, Goldmann S, Hacker HJ, Weber O, Kramer T, et al: Inhibition of hepatitis B virus replication by drug-induced depletion of nucleocapsids. Science 2003;299: 893–896.

23 Gupta S, Rajvanshi P, Sokhi R, et al: Entry and integration of transplanted hepatocytes in rat liver plates occur by disruption of hepatic sinusoidal endothelium. Hepatology 1999;29:509–519.

24 Novacek MJ: Mammalian phylogeny: Shaking the tree. Nature 1992;356:121–125.

25 Walter E, Keist R, Niederost B, Pult I, Blum HE: Hepatitis B virus infection of tupaia hepatocytes in vitro and in vivo. Hepatology 1996;24:1–5.

26 Köck J, Nassal M, MacNelly S, Baumert TF, Blum HE, von Weizsäcker F: Efficient infection of primary tupaia hepatocytes with purified human and woolly monkey hepatitis B virus. J Virol 2001;75:5084–5089.

27 Glebe D, Aliakbari M, Krass P, Knoop EV, Valerius KP, Gerlich WH: Pre-s1 antigen-dependent infection of tupaia hepatocyte cultures with human hepatitis B virus. J Virol 2003;77:9511–9521.

28 Köck J, Baumert TF, Delaney W, Blum HE, von Weizsäcker F: Inhibitory effect of adefovir and lamivudine on the initiation of hepatitis B virus infection in primary tupaia hepatocytes. Hepatology 2003;38:1410–1418.

29 Burda MR, Dandri M, Zuckerman DM, Will H, Toeroek E, Pollok J, Rogiers X, Gocht A, Greten H, Koeck J, Blum HE, von Weizsäcker F, Petersen J: Cryopreserved tupaia hepatocytes can extensively repopulate the liver of uPA/RAG-2 mice: A new and convenient model for hepatitis B virus infection studies and antiviral drug evaluation (abstract). Hepatology 2002;36(suppl):366A.

30 Cantz T, Zuckerman DM, Burda MR, Dandri M, Goricke B, Thalhammer S, Heckl WM, et al: Quantitative gene expression analysis reveals transition of fetal liver progenitor cells to mature hepatocytes after transplantation in uPA/RAG-2 mice. Am J Pathol 2003;162:37–45.

31 Robertson BH, Margolis HS: Primate hepatitis B viruses – Genetic diversity, geography and evolution. Rev Med Virol 2002;12:133–141.

32 Werle B, Wursthorn K, Petersen J, Bowden S, Locarnini S, Lau G, Trepo C, et al: Quantitative analysis of hepatic HBV cccDNA during the natural history of chronic hepatitis B and adefovir dipivoxil therapy: An international, multicenter study (abstract). Hepatology 2002;36(suppl):296A.

33 Fautrel A, Joly B, Guyomard C, Guillouzo A: Long-term maintenance of drug-metabolizing enzyme activities in rat hepatocytes after cryopreservation. Toxicol Appl Pharmacol 1997;147: 110–114.

34 Dandri M, Burda MR, Gocht A, Torok E, Pollok JM, Rogler CE, Will H, Petersen J: Woodchuck hepatocytes remain permissive for hepadnavirus infection and mouse liver repopulation after cryopreservation. Hepatology 2001;34:824–833.
35 Zhao X, Tang ZY, Klumpp B, Wolff-Vorbeck G, Barth H, Levy S, von Weizsäcker F, Blum HE, Baumert TF: Primary hepatocytes of *Tupaia belangeri* as a potential model for hepatitis C virus infection. J Clin Invest 2002;109:221–232.

Maura Dandri
Department of Medicine, University Hospital Hamburg-Eppendorf and
Heinrich-Pette-Institute for Experimental Virology and Immunology
University of Hamburg, DE–20246 Hamburg, Germany
Tel. +49 40 4280 32949, Fax +49 40 4280 37232, E-Mail m.dandri@uke.uni-hamburg.de

von Weizsäcker F, Roggendorf M (eds): Models of Viral Hepatitis.
Monogr Virol. Basel, Karger, 2005, vol 25, pp 146–160

The Trimera Mouse Model of HBV and HCV Infection

Wulf O. Böcher[a], *Yair Reisner*[b]

[a]First Department of Internal Medicine, University of Mainz, Mainz, Germany and [b]Department of Immunology, The Weizmann Institute of Science, Rehovot, Israel

Although the hepatitis B and C virus are similar with regard to clinical manifestations and complications, the lack of cytopathicity, their hepatotropism and parenteral transmission mode, both viruses differ substantially in their potential to induce chronic infection. Moreover, both viruses induce hepatitis by inducing antiviral immune responses that inhibit viral replication via cytopathic and non-cytopathic pathways leading to spontaneous resolution if strong and multispecific Th cell and CTL responses develop, or to chronic viral persistence, if the response is weak and oligospecific [1]. Whereas the innate immune response seems to be important in the early phases of HBV infection [2, 3], the broad and strong antiviral Th cell and CTL response has been shown to be crucial for termination of viral replication and clinical resolution [4]. Moreover, spontaneous or IFN-α-induced resolution from hepatitis B or C is strongly correlated with the development or resurgence of strong antiviral T-cell responses, underlining the importance of the adaptive immune response [5, 6]. Current therapeutic options for both diseases are very limited with the standard course of IFN-α treatment leading to remissions in less than 30% of carefully selected HBV patients and in combination with ribavirin in less than 50% of chronic HCV patients. The nucleoside analogue lamivudine induces a response in a substantial proportion of patients but this effect is transient in the majority of HBV patients due to the rapid emergence of resistance mutants. Similar effects may occur under long-term treatment with adefovir. Thus, new therapeutic options are urgently needed, taking into account the high prevalence of both infections in western countries and worldwide.

Due to the striking differences in strength and multispecificity of the antiviral immune responses in chronic as compared to resolving patients, it is tempting to speculate that increasing the antiviral responses of chronic carriers might lead to viral elimination or clinical resolution. Thus, two ways of immunostimulation have been studied for HBV infection: adoptive transfer of anti-HBV immunity by stem cell transplantation [7] and therapeutic vaccination. In 80% of chronic HBV patients who for hematological malignancies received HLA-matched bone marrow from donors who had spontaneously resolved from HBV infection before, bone marrow reconstitution led to resolution from hepatitis B [7, 8]. Since HBs vaccination of donors before donation of the bone marrow was not sufficient to induce resolution from hepatitis B, it was speculated that HBc-specific T cells that were demonstrated in donors and recipients were crucial for the antiviral activity of the graft [8]. However, bone marrow transplantation is obviously not a therapeutic option for the vast majority of patients with chronic HBV or HCV infection, and therefore therapeutic vaccination with envelope antigens or the immunodominant core-derived CTL epitope HBc_{18-27} has been studied in clinical trials. The preS/S vaccine used by the French group did induce strong HBs and preS-specific antibody and Th cell responses in healthy vaccinees, but only rare T-cell proliferative responses limited to the original vaccine and no relevant virological responses were found in chronic HBV patients [9, 10]. Similarly, vaccination with the modified peptide vaccine induced specific CTL responses in healthy volunteers but not in patients, corresponding to a lack of virological or biochemical responses [11].

Although the rationale for therapeutic vaccination for HCV infection in principle would be the same, no clinical data have been published yet. However, vaccination for hepatitis C as compared to hepatitis B is strongly hampered by the high genetic variability of the virus leading to a large number of different HCV genotypes and subtypes. Moreover, within an infected individual the virus exists as a quasispecies underlying a dynamic process of genetic alterations leading to the rapid emergence of immunological escape mutants. Thus, a candidate vaccine would either have to consist of highly conserved but nevertheless immunogenic antigens or have to consider the genotype and the mutational status of the infecting virus in each individual patient.

Thus, although the proof of principle of a therapeutic effect of antiviral immunostimulation has been demonstrated by adoptive transfer experiments, the more widely applicable way of therapeutic vaccination has been unsuccessful due to the yet undefined immune failure of chronic patients. In order to assess further vaccine candidates in a preclinical setting, the humanized trimera mouse model was established that allowed to transfer the immune defect from the patient into the mouse by transplantation of patient PBMC. A vaccine that under these conditions would stimulate strong and multispecific patient T-cell responses and exert antiviral effects would be expected to have a high chance of being efficient in human studies as well.

The Humanized Trimera Mouse Model

The major obstacle for research on HBV and HCV infection is the lack of a suitable small animal model due to the host specificity of both viruses. However, the species specificity of the virus can be broken by implantation of human tissues into susceptible mice. Such a humanized model of immunotherapeutic interventions should support viremia as well as engraftment of a functioning immune system in an autologous setting. The most commonly used humanized mouse model in the early 1990s employed mice with severe combined immunodeficiency (scid) as recipients for human tissues and PBMC [12]. These mice have a congenital defect of nuclear recombinases and are unable to recombine specific B- and T-cell receptors and therefore lack any specific B and T cells leading to immunological ignorance of allo- or xenoreactive tissues. These mice were implanted with human tissues such as thymus, spleen, PBMC or human tumors and did facilitate a transient engraftment of the respective tissues allowing limited studies of human diseases such as HIV infection as well as vaccination studies [13]. However, due to their slow engraftment, human B and T cells recovered from such mice at the time of peak engraftment were anergic [14]. Only very early after PBMC transfer could functional antigen-specific T cells be isolated in very low numbers from PBL-scid mice, strongly limiting this model for immunological studies [15].

In contrast to these congenitally immunodeficient mice, trimera mice have been shown to support rapid engraftment of transferred PBMC resulting in a well-preserved function of transferred B and T cells. This model employs Balb/c mice that undergo lethal split-dose total body irradiation and transplantation of scid mouse bone marrow for reconstitution with erythroid and myeloid lineages [16] (fig. 1). Such mice can then receive human liver tissue implants under the kidney capsule leading to functional and structural engraftment of this tissue for a period of several weeks to months. The term trimera is derived from its three components, the Balb/c recipient, the scid mouse bone marrow donor and the human PBMC or tissue donor. If the implanted human liver tissue is infected by HBV or HCV (in vivo or in vitro), the recipient mice become viremic [17–21]. Alternatively, high numbers of human PBMC can be transferred intraperitoneally resulting in a transient reconstitution of the mouse for a period of more than 4 weeks [16]. Thymectomy of recipient mice several weeks before implantation led to a further increase of engraftment.

The rapid engraftment of human PBMC or tissues results in a number of important functional advantages over the conventional scid mouse models: (1) As a consequence of the rapid engraftment of transferred PBMC occurring within days after transfer [16], human lymphocytes can be recovered from peritoneum, spleen and other tissues at very early time points, before xenoreactivity

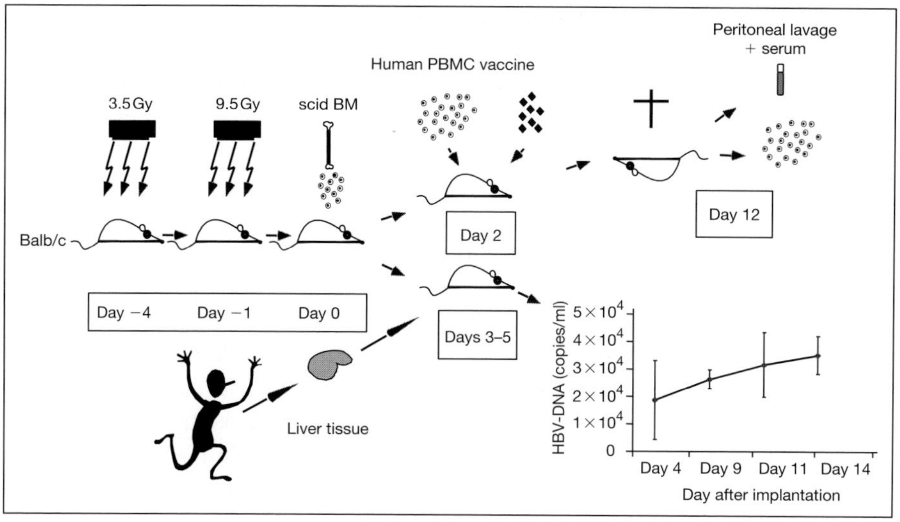

Fig. 1. The trimera mouse model.

leads to anergy of transferred human Th cells or CTL. Thus, primary and memory antibody, Th cell and CTL responses can be induced in vivo and detected ex vivo [22–24]. The high speed human lymphocyte engraftment is believed to be the resultant of the high cell numbers being transferred and the preexistence of lymphoid organs in the recipient mouse [25]. (2) Human lymphoid follicle-like structures are detectable in the Balb/c host with human B and T cells residing in close proximity [26]. This structurally overt engraftment is thought to be due to the preexistence of lymphoid organs in irradiated Balb/c recipients and interspecies cross-reactivity of murine and human lymphocyte homing factors. (3) Possibly as a consequence of this functionally active human immune system, extraordinarily high numbers of human PBMC up to 10^8/mouse can be transferred into trimera mice without induction of EBV lymphomas [27–29]. (4) As a possible consequence of the preserved function and low xenoreactivity of transferred human T cells, the rate of clinically relevant graft-versus-host disease is negligible in trimera mice despite the high numbers of transferred PBMC [16]. (5) Finally, in principle any mouse with a given genetic background can be humanized using the trimera approach [25]. Thus, by the use of genetically modified recipient mice the transplanted PBMC or tissue could be modified in vivo to study the influence of a transgene or knockout gene on the respective tissue.

These structural advantages of the trimera over the scid and $rag^{-/-}$ mouse models are reflected by the enhanced function of the transferred human immune system. In a head-to-head comparison between human/Balb/c and human/cb17.scid chimera, antigen-specific antibody responses were significantly higher in the former mice [23]. Moreover, primary antigen-specific human Th cell and CTL responses were induced in trimera mice [22, 24], whereas transferred human B and T cells recovered at the peak of engraftment from scid chimera occurring as late as 4–8 weeks after PBMC transfer are severely dysfunctional due to severe limitations of the transferred B- and T-cell receptor repertoire, anergy and xenoreactivity [30–33]. Only when recovered from scid mice at very early time points after PBMC transfer could memory T-cell responses be detected in one study, although cell numbers were very low and had to be pooled from several mice [15]. Rag-1- or -2-deficient mice sharing the phenotype with scid mice showed a significantly weaker engraftment and antibody production than scid mice when used as PBMC and vaccine recipients [34]. Thus, these mice have widely been abandoned as models for human diseases or vaccination studies since the late 1990s, while the trimera mouse has proven useful in recent years to generate clinically active human monoclonal antibodies against HBV and HCV [21, 35, 36], to study embryonic immunogenicity [37] and as model to study immunopathogenesis and immunotherapy of chronic B-lymphocytic leukemia [38, 39] or human viral infections such as influenza, HBV, HCV and HIV infection [17–22, 40–42].

HBV/HCV Replication in the Trimera

The trimera model supports the engraftment of any xenogeneic tissue, such as human liver tissue, under the murine kidney capsule that is chosen as the preferred site of implantation for two reasons: (1) the rapid de novo development of blood vessels out of the kidney capsule provides the implant with excellent nutrition and (2) the implant is fixed firmly under the kidney capsule and can therefore easily be refound after various periods of time for histological or other studies. Although some fibrosis is usually found 4 weeks after implantation, the typical hepatic architecture of the implant is quite well preserved until that time (fig. 2). The engraftment rate after 1 month approximates 85% and the viability of hepatocytes was demonstrated by the expression of human serum albumin mRNA in the implants [20].

The model was originally established as a small animal model to study HCV infection [18]. BNX mice were employed as recipients for subrenocapsular implantation of HCV-infected human liver tissue, leading in these first experiments to a temporary liver engraftment, with approximately 50% of implanted trimera mice developing HCV viremia detectable by RT-PCR. After implantation of ex vivo infected human liver tissue, only 25% of recipient mice became viremic. Later on, these studies were extended using thymectomized

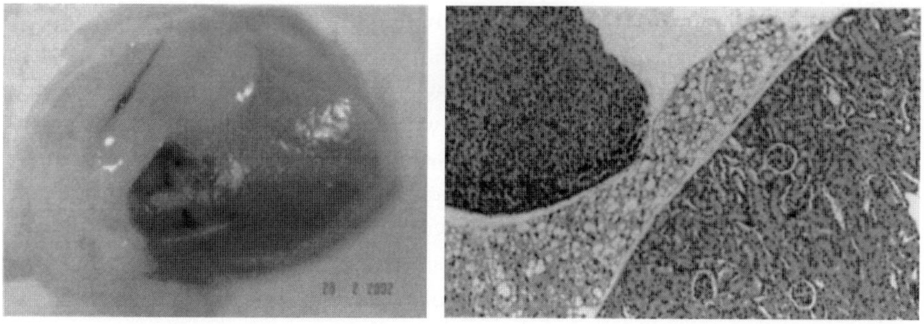

a *b*

Fig. 2. Trimera kidney with subcapsular human liver tissue from a patient with chronic active HBV infection explanted 10 days after implantation. ***a*** ×25, ***b*** HE staining, ×200.

CB6 mice, irradiated according to an optimized split radiation protocol, as recipients of in vivo or ex vivo infected human liver tissues [21]. The surgery-related mortality of recipient mice was 15–25% and the peak of HCV viremia was reached 18–20 days after implantation with 85% of recipients being viremic. The peak levels reached in trimera mice were 1.5×10^4 up to 1×10^5 copies/ml, whether the implant was infected ex vivo or obtained from a patient. Immediately after implantation, virus was detectable in serum, dropped over the next few days and then steadily increased together with an increase of minus-strand RNA as the replicative intermediate, reaching a peak on day 20 after implantation. After that time point, viral RNA levels progressively decreased and finally became undetectable between 25 and 34 days after implantation due to progressive fibrosis and necrosis of the liver implant [21]. Importantly, HCV viremia could therapeutically be modified by application of a new antiviral compound or a monoclonal anti-HCV antibody, demonstrating the suitability of this model for evaluation of antiviral therapy.

After infection of healthy human liver tissue ex vivo with high-titer HBV serum followed by subrenocapsular implantation, up to 80% of recipient mice were progressively infected, developing peak HBV viremia 18–20 days after implantation. As in the HCV-trimera model, viremia dropped over the following weeks reaching undetectable levels 45–50 days after implantation. The presence of IL-6 seemed to play an important role during this in vitro infection process [17]. The kinetics of viremia as well as the demonstration of HBV-derived rcDNA and cccDNA in the implants excluded a mere contamination of the mice with non-replicative HBV [17, 20]. Moreover, as after HCV infection, the percentage of HBV-infected animals as well as the mean viral load of the animals could therapeutically be modified by administration of antivirals such as lamivudine or anti-HBs antibodies to the mice [20]. Subrenocapsular implantation of liver tissue generated from diagnostic liver punctures of chronic HBV patients did induce HBV viremia in trimera recipients with similar kinetics (fig. 1, 2). Thus, although the window of liver engraftment and viremia is currently limited to approximately 4–5 weeks, the trimera mouse provides a model supporting full HBV and HCV viral replication that can be therapeutically modified.

Induction and Characterization of Human Immune Responses in the Trimera

The principle idea of producing human/Balb/scid chimeric mice was to generate a model for studies of the human immune system, hematopoiesis, autoimmunity, malignant or infectious diseases in any mouse with a given genetic background. However, the major point of interest rapidly became the transfer of a functioning immune system from human to mouse, opening the possibility to induce and study antigen-specific immune responses.

Marcus et al. [23] demonstrated that in vivo vaccination of trimera reconstituted with PBMC from healthy vaccinated or immunized donors led to strong anti-tetanus or anti-HBs antibody responses. In addition to these recall responses, strong primary antibody responses against keyhole limpet hemocyanin (KLH) and the recombinant HIV-derived protein nef could be induced in vivo leading to an IgM/IgG isotype shift of the specific antibody response. The magnitude and quality of these anti-KLH antibody responses in trimera mice was significantly superior to that in conventional scid mice. Whereas T cells recovered from scid mice are dysfunctional as stated above, the assessment of T-cell function of human PBMC recovered 12–30 days after transfer from peritoneum and spleen of trimera mice revealed strong proliferative responses to OKT-3 and IL-2 [24]. Moreover, specific CTL against allogeneic target and Raji tumor cells could be induced by in vivo vaccination that were demonstrated ex vivo by ^{51}Cr-release assays and in vivo by rejection of the respective tumor implants. Moreover, vaccination of trimera mice with recombinant vaccinia vectors expressing the HIV nef protein resulted in the induction of nef-specific CTL demonstrated by ^{51}Cr-release assays [24]. Recently, a marked effect of vaccination against influenza could be obtained by intranasal administration of the antigen, further demonstrating that human responses are not limited to the peritoneal site of lymphocyte infusion [40]. Studies of the kinetics of the developing antigen-specific B- and T-cell responses in the trimera revealed a functional peak engraftment as early as 10–15 days after PBMC transfer [43]. More recent studies could confirm the successful induction of primary and secondary antigen-specific Th cell and CTL responses

In contrast, the trimera model in its current form provides a window of functional engraftment of xenotransplanted liver tissue or PBMC limited to a maximum of 4–6 weeks, that might possibly be increased by substitution of growth factors, such as the described cMet-agonistic antibody. However, similar levels of viremia can be achieved in this model by implantation of HBV- or HCV-infected liver tissue obtained by diagnostic needle biopsy without the need of isolating hepatocytes. Moreover, the trimera is the only model with well-documented functional engraftment of PBMC enabling studies of immunotherapeutic interventions [36].

Conclusion

The trimera model has proven useful to assess human vaccine responses in vivo and to support replication of human-specific viruses such as HBV and HCV. Thus, it is suitable for studies of virus replication or antivirals. Since the peak engraftment of liver tissue and PBMC simultaneously occurs within 4 weeks after transplant, a therapeutic effect of an immunogenic vaccine on the amount of viremia after combined implantation of autologous PBMC and liver tissue from HBV patients is anticipated. Further studies are directed towards defining a candidate vaccine with the potential to induce strong anti-HBs antibody and antiviral Th cell and CTL responses.

References

1 Bertoletti A, Ferrari C: Kinetics of the immune response during HBV and HCV infection. Hepatology 2003;38:4–13.

2 Guidotti LG, Rochford R, Chung J, Shapiro M, Purcell R, Chisari FV: Viral clearance without destruction of infected cells during acute HBV infection. Science 1999;284:825–829.

3 Webster GJ, Reignat S, Maini MK, Whalley SA, Ogg GS, King A, Brown D, Amlot PL, Williams R, Vergani D, Dusheiko GM, Bertoletti A: Incubation phase of acute hepatitis B in man: Dynamic of cellular immune mechanisms. Hepatology 2000;32:1117–1124.

4 Thimme R, Wieland S, Steiger C, Ghrajeb J, Reimann KA, Purcell RH, Chisari FV: CD8(+) T cells mediate viral clearance and disease pathogenesis during acute hepatitis B virus infection. J Virol 2002;77:68–76.

5 Tsai SL, Chen PJ, Lai MY, Yang PM, Sung JL, Huang JH, Hwang LH, Chang TH, Chen DS: Acute exacerbations of chronic type B hepatitis are accompanied by increased T cell responses to hepatitis B core and e antigens. Implications for hepatitis B e antigen seroconversion. J Clin Invest 1992;89:87–96.

6 Löhr HF, Gerken G, Roth M, Weyer S, Schlaak JF, Meyer zum Büschenfelde KH: The cellular immune responses induced in the follow-up of interferon-α-treated patients with chronic hepatitis C may determine the therapy outcome. J Hepatol 1998;29:524–532.

7 Ilan Y, Nagler A, Adler R, Tur KR, Slavin S, Shouval D: Ablation of persistent hepatitis B by bone marrow transplantation from a hepatitis B-immune donor. Gastroenterology 1993;104: 1818–1821.

8 Lau GK, Suri D, Liang R, Rigopoulou E, Thomas M, Mullerova I, Nanji A, Yuen ST, Williams R, Naoumov N: Resolution of chronic hepatitis B and anti-HBs seroconversion in humans by adoptive transfer of immunity to hepatitis B core antigen. Gastroenterology 2002;122:614–624.

9 Couillin I, Pol S, Mancini M, Driss F, Brechot C, Tiollais P, Michel ML: Specific vaccine therapy in chronic hepatitis B: Induction of T cell proliferative responses specific for envelope antigens. J Infect Dis 1999;180:15–26.

10 Pol S, Nalpas B, Driss F, Michel ML, Tiollais P, Denis J, Brechot C: Efficacy and limitations of a specific immunotherapy in chronic hepatitis B. J Hepatol 2001;34:917–921.

11 Heathcote J, McHutchison J, Lee S, Tong M, Benner K, Minuk G, Wright T, Fikes J, Livingston B, Sette A, Chestnut R: A pilot study of the CY-1899 T-cell vaccine in subjects chronically infected with hepatitis B virus. Hepatology 1999;30:531–536.

12 Bosma GC, Custer RP, Bosma MJ: A severe combined immunodeficiency mutation in the mouse. Nature 1983;301:527–530.

13 Mosier DE, Gulizia RJ, Baird SM, Wilson DB: Transfer of a functional human immune system to mice with severe combined immunodeficiency. Nature 1988;335:256–259.

14 Tary Lehmann M, Saxon A, Lehmann PV: The human immune system in hu-PBL-SCID mice. Immunol Today 1995;16:529–533.

15 Albert SE, McKerlie C, Pester A, Edgell BJ, Carlyle J, Petric M, Chamberlain JW: Time-dependent induction of protective anti-influenza immune responses in human peripheral blood lymphocyte/SCID mice. J Immunol 1997;159:1393–1403.

16 Lubin I, Segall H, Marcus H, David M, Kulova L, Steinitz M, Erlich P, Gan J, Reisner Y: Engraftment of human peripheral blood lymphocytes in normal strains of mice. Blood 1994; 83:2368–2381.

17 Galun E, Nahor O, Eid A, Jurim O, Rose-John S, Blum HE, Nussbaum O, Ilan E, Daudi N, Shouval D, Reisner Y, Dagan S: Human interleukin-6 facilitates hepatitis B virus infection in vitro and in vivo. Virology 2000;270:299–309.

18 Galun E, Burakova T, Ketzinel M, Lubin I, Shezen E, Kahana Y, Eid A, Ilan Y, Rivkind A, Pizov G, et al: Hepatitis C virus viremia in SCID→BNX mouse chimera. J Infect Dis 1995;172:25–30.

19 Ilan E, Burakova T, Dagan S, Nussbaum O, Lubin I, Eren R, Ben-Moshe O, Arazi J, Berr S, Neville L, Yuen L, Mansour TS, Gillard J, Eid A, Jurim O, Shouval D, Reisner Y, Galun E: The HBV-trimera mouse: A model for human HBV infection and evaluation of anti-HBV therapeutic agents. Hepatology 1999;29:553–562.

20 Ilan E, Burakova T, Dagan S, Nussbaum O, Lubin I, Eren R, Ben-Moshe O, Arazi J, Berr S, Neville L, Yuen L, Mansour TS, Gillard J, Eid A, Jurim O, Shouval D, Reisner Y, Galun E: The hepatitis B virus-trimera mouse: A model for human HBV infection and evaluation of anti-HBV therapeutic agents. Hepatology 1999;29:553–562.

21 Ilan E, Arazi J, Nussbaum O, Zauberman A, Eren R, Lubin I, Neville L, Ben-Moshe O, Kischitzky A, Litchi A, Margalit I, Gopher J, Mounir S, Cai W, Daudi N, Eid A, Jurim O, Czerniak A, Galun E, Dagan S: The hepatitis C virus (HCV)-trimera mouse: A model for evaluation of agents against HCV. J Infect Dis 2002;185:153–161.

22 Böcher W, Dekel B, Schwerin W, Geissler M, Hoffmann S, Rohwer A, Arditti F, Cooper A, Bernhard H, Berrebi A, Rose-John S, Shaul Y, Galle PR, Loehr HF, Reisner Y: Induction of strong hepatitis B virus (HBV) specific T helper cell and cytotoxic T lymphocyte responses by therapeutic vaccination in the trimera mouse model of chronic HBV infection. Eur J Immunol 2001;31:2071–2079.

23 Marcus H, David M, Canaan A, Kulova L, Lubin I, Segall H, Denes L, Erlich P, Galun E, Gan J, Reisner Y: Human/mouse radiation chimera are capable of mounting a human primary humoral response. Blood 1995;86:398–406.

24 Segall H, Lubin I, Marcus H, Canaan A, Reisner Y: Generation of primary antigen-specific human cytotoxic T lymphocytes in human/mouse radiation chimera. Blood 1996;88:721–730.

25 Reisner Y, Dagan S: The trimera mouse: A novel system for the generation of human monoclonal antibodies and models for human diseases. Trends Biotechnol 1998;16:242–246.

26 Burakova T, Marcus H, Canaan A, Dekel B, Shezen E, David M, Lubin I, Segal H, Reisner Y: Engrafted human T and B lymphocytes form mixed follicles in lymphoid organs of human/mouse and human/rat chimera. Transplantation 1997;63:1166–1171.

27 Marcus H, Burakova T, Shezen E, David M, Canaan A, Lubin I, Reisner Y: Human→mouse radiation chimera do not develop Epstein-Barr virus lymphoma. Immunol Lett 1996;49:155–161.
28 Rowe M, Young LS, Crocker J, Stokes H, Henderson S, Rickinson AB: Epstein-Barr virus (EBV)-associated lymphoproliferative disease in the SCID mouse model: Implications for the pathogenesis of EBV-positive lymphomas in man. J Exp Med 1991;173:147–158.
29 Wagar EJ, Cromwell MA, Shultz LD, Woda BA, Sullivan JL, Hesselton RM, Greiner DL: Regulation of human cell engraftment and development of EBV-related lymphoproliferative disorders in Hu-PBL-scid mice. J Immunol 2000;165:518–527.
30 Tary Lehmann M, Saxon A: Human mature T cells that are anergic in vivo prevail in SCID mice reconstituted with human peripheral blood. J Exp Med 1992;175:503–516.
31 Tary Lehmann M, Lehmann PV, Schols D, Roncarolo MG, Saxon A: Anti-SCID mouse reactivity shapes the human CD4+ T cell repertoire in hu-PBL-SCID chimeras. J Exp Med 1994;180: 1817–1827.
32 Saxon A, Macy E, Denis K, Tary Lehmann M, Witte O, Braun J: Limited B cell repertoire in severe combined immunodeficient mice engrafted with peripheral blood mononuclear cells derived from immunodeficient or normal humans. J Clin Invest 1991;87:658–665.
33 Garcia S, Dadaglio G, Gougeon ML: Limits of the human-PBL-SCID mice model: Severe restriction of the V β T-cell repertoire of engrafted human T cells. Blood 1997;89:329–336.
34 Steinsvik TE, Gaarder PI, Aaberge IS, Lovik M: Engraftment and humoral immunity in SCID and RAG-2-deficient mice transplanted with human peripheral blood lymphocytes. Scand J Immunol 1995;42:607–616.
35 Eren R, Lubin I, Terkieltaub D, Ben-Moshe O, Zauberman A, Uhlman R, Tzahor T, Moss S, Ilan E, Shouval D, Galun E, Daudi N, Marcus H, Reisner Y, Dagan S: Human monoclonal antibodies specific to hepatitis B virus generated in a human/mouse radiation chimera: The trimera system. Immunology 1998;93:154–161.
36 Eren R, Ilan E, Nussbaum O, Lubin I, Terkieltaub D, Arazi Y, Ben-Moshe O, Kitchinzky A, Berr S, Gopher J, Zauberman A, Galun E, Shouval D, Daudi N, Eid A, Jurim O, Magnius LO, Hammas B, Reisner Y, Dagan S: Preclinical evaluation of two human anti-hepatitis B virus (HBV) monoclonal antibodies in the HBV-trimera mouse model and in HBV chronic carrier chimpanzees. Hepatology 2000;32:588–596.
37 Dekel B, Burakova T, Arditti FD, Reich-Zeliger S, Milstein O, Aviel-Ronen S, Rechavi G, Friedman N, Kaminski N, Passwell JH, Reisner Y: Human and porcine early kidney precursors as a new source for transplantation. Nat Med 2003;9:53–60.
38 Shimoni A, Marcus H, Canaan A, Ergas D, David M, Berrebi A, Reisner Y: A model for human B-chronic lymphocytic leukemia in human/mouse radiation chimera: Evidence for tumor-mediated suppression of antibody production in low-stage disease. Blood 1997;89:2210–2218.
39 Shimoni A, Marcus H, Dekel B, Shkarchi R, Arditti F, Shvidel L, Shtalrid M, Böcher W, Canaan A, Ergas D, Berrebi A, Reisner Y: Autologous T cells control B-chronic lymphocytic leukemia tumor progression in human→mouse radiation chimera. Cancer Res 1999;59:5968–5974.
40 Ben-Yedidia T, Marcus H, Reisner Y, Arnon R: Intranasal administration of peptide vaccine protects human/mouse radiation chimera from influenza infection. Int Immunol 1999;11:1043–1051.
41 Böcher WO, Galun E, Marcus H, Daudi N, Terkieltaub D, Shouval D, Löhr HF, Reisner Y: Reduced hepatitis B virus surface antigen-specific Th1 helper cell frequency of chronic HBV Carriers is associated with a failure to produce antigen-specific antibodies in human/mouse radiation chimera. Hepatology 2000;31:480–487.
42 Shapira-Nahor O, Marcus H, Segall H, Lubin I, Slavin S, Panet A, Reisner Y: Human T cells recovered from human/Balb radiation chimeras are hypersensitive to human immunodeficiency virus type 1 infection. J Virol 1997;71:4495–4501.
43 Böcher WO, Marcus H, Shakarchy R, Dekel B, Galun E, Reisner Y: Antigen specific B and T cells in the human/mouse radiation chimera following immunization in vivo. Immunology 1999; 96:634–641.
44 Jung MC, Diepolder HM, Spengler U, Wierenga EA, Zachoval R, Hoffmann RM, Eichenlaub D, Frosner G, Will H, Pape GR: Activation of a heterogeneous hepatitis B (HB) core and e antigen-specific CD4+ T-cell population during seroconversion to anti-HBe and anti-HBs in hepatitis B virus infection. J Virol 1995;69:3358–3368.

45 Löhr HF, Weber W, Schlaak J, Goergen B, Meyer zum Büschenfelde KH, Gerken G: Proliferative response of CD4+ T cells and hepatitis B virus clearance in chronic hepatitis with or without hepatitis B e-minus hepatitis B virus mutants. Hepatology 1995;22:61–68.

46 Ferrari C, Penna A, Bertoletti A, Valli A, Antoni AD, Giuberti T, Cavalli A, Petit MA, Fiaccadori F: Cellular immune response to hepatitis B virus-encoded antigens in acute and chronic hepatitis B virus infection. J Immunol 1990;145:3442–3449.

47 Penna A, Artini M, Cavalli A, Levrero M, Bertoletti A, Pilli M, Chisari FV, Rehermann B, Del Prete G, Fiaccadori F, Ferrari C: Long-lasting memory T cell responses following self-limited acute hepatitis B. J Clin Invest 1996;98:1185–1194.

48 Rehermann B, Ferrari C, Pasquinelli C, Chisari FV: The hepatitis B virus persists for decades after patients' recovery from acute viral hepatitis despite active maintenance of a cytotoxic T-lymphocyte response. Nat Med 1996;2:1104–1108.

49 Kock J, Schlicht HJ: Analysis of the earliest steps of hepadnavirus replication: Genome repair after infectious entry into hepatocytes does not depend on viral polymerase activity. J Virol 1993;67:4867–4874.

50 Lu M, Hilken G, Kruppenbacher J, Kemper T, Schirmbeck R, Reimann J, Roggendorf M: Immunization of woodchucks with plasmids expressing woodchuck hepatitis virus (WHV) core antigen and surface antigen suppresses WHV infection. J Virol 1999;73:281–289.

51 Bassett S, Guerra B, Brasky K, Miskovsky E, Houghton M, Klimpel GR, Lanford RE: Protective immune response to hepatitis C virus in chimpanzees rechallenged following clearance of primary infection. Hepatology 2001;33:1479–1487.

52 Chisari FV: Hepatitis B virus transgenic mice: Insights into the virus and the disease. Hepatology 1995;22:1316–1325.

53 Petersen J, Dandri M, Gupta S, Rogler CE: Liver repopulation with xenogenic hepatocytes in B and T cell-deficient mice leads to chronic hepadnavirus infection and clonal growth of hepatocellular carcinoma. Proc Natl Acad Sci USA 1998;95:310–315.

54 Ohashi K, Marion PL, Nakai H, Meuse L, Cullen JM, Bordier BB, Schwall R, Greenberg HB, Glenn JS, Kay MA: Sustained survival of human hepatocytes in mice: A model for in vivo infection with human hepatitis B and hepatitis δ viruses. Nat Med 2000;6:327–331.

55 Mercer DF, Schiller DE, Elliott JF, Douglas DN, Hao C, Rinfret A, Kneteman NM: Hepatitis C virus replication in mice with chimeric human livers. Nat Med 2001;7:927–933.

Wulf O. Böcher, MD
First Department of Internal Medicine, Johannes Gutenberg University
Langenbeckstrasse 1, DE–55131 Mainz (Germany)
Tel. +49 6131 172666, Fax +49 6131 176621
E-Mail boecher@mail.uni-mainz.de

Subject Index